THE SARS EPIDEMIC

Challenges to China's Crisis Management

THE SARS EPIDEMIC

Challenges to China's Crisis Management

editors

John Wong
Zheng Yongnian
East Asian Institute, National University of Singapore

World Scientific
NEW JERSEY • LONDON • SINGAPORE • BEIJING • SHANGHAI • HONG KONG • TAIPEI • CHENNAI

Published by

World Scientific Publishing Co. Pte. Ltd.
5 Toh Tuck Link, Singapore 596224
USA office: Suite 202, 1060 Main Street, River Edge, NJ 07661
UK office: 57 Shelton Street, Covent Garden, London WC2H 9HE

British Library Cataloguing-in-Publication Data
A catalogue record for this book is available from the British Library.

THE SARS EPIDEMIC: CHALLENGES TO CHINA'S CRISIS MANAGEMENT

ISBN 981-238-948-2

Typeset by Stallion Press
E-mail: sales@stallionpress.com

Printed in Singapore by World Scientific Printers (S) Pte Ltd

Contents

Editors

John WONG, Research Director, East Asian Institute
ZHENG Yongnian, Senior Research Fellow, East Asian Institute

Contributors

CAO Cong, Research Fellow, East Asian Institute
Sarah CHAN, Research Officer, East Asian Institute
GU Xin, Professor, Beijing Normal University
HE Baogang, Senior Research Fellow, East Asian Institute
LAI Hongyi, Research Fellow, East Asian Institute
LIANG Ruobing, Research Officer, East Asian Institute
LYE Liang Fook, Research Officer, East Asian Institute
Elspeth THOMSON, Research Fellow, East Asian Institute
YOW Cheun Hoe, Research Officer, East Asian Institute
ZOU Keyuan, Senior Research Fellow, East Asian Institute

SARS and Governance in China

JOHN WONG AND ZHENG YONGNIAN

In the first half of 2003, severe acute respiratory syndrome (SARS) suddenly struck China and Hong Kong, claiming many lives and causing panic. It also jolted their economic growth, disrupted the social life of their citizens, and created much stress and strain on their political systems and governance.

Like dealing with other "external shocks", the management of the SARS crisis provides a good opportunity to examine the weaknesses and strengths of the political systems of China and its special administrative area, Hong Kong. Although both are Chinese communities, their political systems differ. China remains an authoritarian political system, despite the dramatic economic transformation that has occurred over the past two decades. Hong Kong inherited the British colonial political system with a rich tradition of rule of law and an efficient bureaucracy. Nevertheless, after its return to China, societal demands for greater democratization have increased. Given the different political settings of these two Chinese communities, it would be interesting to examine how they responded to the SARS crisis.

From the outset, scholars at the East Asian Institute (EAI) have followed closely the unfolding of SARS events in China and Hong Kong, particularly how each of the two societies has come to grips with such a "random shock". SARS may or may not recur in the near future, and many of its effects may only be short-term in nature. However, the episode has produced some long-term structural consequences. In particular, it offers a good glimpse of the relative resilience of the two societies, the quality of their respective political leadership, the effectiveness of their political and institutional mobilization, the crisis-management capability of their respective bureaucracies, and the viability of their governance systems.

This volume is the result of an EAI workshop on "SARS in China: Crises and Responses" in November 2003. Contributors to this volume are EAI scholars and visiting fellows. Each scholar was asked to contribute a paper to the workshop based on his/her own area of expertise. After intensive discussions during the workshop, each paper underwent further revision for this publication. This volume is organized in the following way. The first chapter provides a comprehensive overview of the impact of the SARS crisis in China and Hong Kong. In doing so, the authors also briefly cover Taiwan's economy. The next six chapters examine the development of the SARS crisis in China from different perspectives. The last chapter discusses SARS in Hong Kong.

THE ECONOMIC IMPACT

The SARS not only caused hundreds of lives, but also affected different economies. In their paper, Wong, Chan and Liang give an overall view of the economic impact of the SARS. They found that the impact operated like a cyclical phenomenon, disrupting economic growth much akin to a business cycle affecting both the demand and supply sides in the short run. The demand shock to the economy was reflected by a fall in consumption. From the supply side, the SARS disrupted production and business operations, which adversely affected the services, particularly the travel industries, and certain manufacturing industries in the SARS affected region. Trade was also hampered, aggravating the supply-side shocks. The negative external shock of SARS further manifested itself through the financial markets, as market confidence weakened and stock prices fell.

Apart from the "cyclical effects", the SARS crisis also exposed or perpetuated the structural weaknesses of the economies, for instance, the high structural unemployment, budget deficits and persistent deflation. Measures to cope with the outbreak of SARS also entailed substantial fiscal costs, including increased expenditures for upgrading medical capabilities and financial assistance to cushion the economic fallout of the outbreak. The fiscal implication was most significant for Hong Kong where its fiscal position was already weak compared to its neighbors like China and Taiwan.

Nevertheless, the three authors also observed that the strong economic fundamentals of the Greater China economies helped them to weather external shocks. China, Hong Kong and Taiwan were able to withstand the fallout from the SARS in varying degrees. For China, SARS did not much dent its economic growth. China has a huge continental economy driven by domestic sources of growth and is thus better able to absorb external shocks compared to other smaller economies like Hong Kong and Singapore.

For Taiwan whose economy was already slowing down before the SARS crisis, the effects of SARS appeared to be short-lived as the economy bounced back to respectable growth underpinned by a moderate recovery in exports and industrial production. Hong Kong was the worst hit compared to China and Taiwan. The SARS dealt a double whammy to its economy which was already mired in recession before the crisis occurred. Lost revenue from tourism further compounded the weak local consumption expenditure and exacerbated the already worsening unemployment situation. Even when the SARS was brought under control, economic recovery at best remained weak, incipient and fragile as Hong Kong continued to be plagued by persistent deflation, serious structural unemployment and high budget deficit. On the whole, the Greater China economies have been resilient even with the occurrence of SARS, as witnessed by a rebound in growth in these economies. Based on their analysis, the three authors concluded that the SARS outbreak has been an exogenous factor that has only limited impact on the Greater China economies in the short-term.

SARS in China

The SARS provides a good example to show how different political systems respond and manage a sudden social crisis. This is especially true in the case of China given the country's size and complexity. In their paper,

Zheng and Lye provide an in-depth analysis of how SARS spread from China to other parts of the world and how the Chinese government responded to the SARS crisis. Initially, China adopted a rather laid-back and disconcerting approach in coping with SARS. It was initially regarded as a purely medical issue which was thought to be best left to local governments or relevant central bureaucratic agencies to handle. It was only when SARS made its presence felt in other parts of the world and international pressures mounted that China began to put its act together.

Nevertheless, Zheng and Lye also pointed out that it would be rather unfair to lay the blame for the spread of SARS squarely on China's failure to institute sufficient preventive measures. The SARS was an entirely new disease. It caught the entire medical community unawares, as nobody fully understood its nature and method of transmission. It would therefore be worthwhile to look beyond the surface and examine the underlying factors that led to China's initial lackluster response. To arrive at a balanced view of how the SARS crisis was managed, Zheng and Lye contends that it is important first to understand the prevailing political context in which the SARS crisis first broke out and China's usual way of handling unpleasant events or news. This could better explain the initial reaction of the Chinese authorities to the outbreak of the disease.

On the one hand, SARS brought out the inherent weaknesses of China's political system in terms of its bureaucratic fragmentation, the delicate nature of China's central-local relations and its civilian-military relations, and the gaping urban-rural divide. On the other hand, SARS also highlighted the internal strengths and resilience of China's political system. The system was still capable of marshaling the necessary resources to curb the spread of the disease once the central authorities had set its focus on the crisis. While identifying the weaknesses and strengths of China's political system, the authors found that leadership matters in coping with the SARS crisis. Hu Jintao and Wen Jiabao were instrumental in mobilizing resources to deal with the problem.

While Zheng and Lye provides an overall view on the political causes of the spread of SARS, Lai examines the issue in detail from the perspective of China's central-local relations. According to Lai, the asymmetric information flow between the localities and the central state posed an institutional problem in the management of SARS. Local bureaucrats and officials have an incentive to distort or suppress negative information from the central government in order to protect their own interests. In this case, Guangdong authorities were very concerned about the potential negative media publicity if news about SARS were made known since this would curtail the domestic spending of the residents, adversely affecting the economic growth of the province and the careers and political fortunes of the local cadres.

Furthermore, communication between localities within the province (e.g., Guangdong) is also seriously insufficient. Some localities like Zhongshan and Guangzhou (two cities in Guangdong Province) were not able to take effective measures against the infectious disease due to lack of first-hand information in Heyuan, where the first case of SARS was reported. Furthermore, there was a lack of information sharing between the military and civilian hospitals. Public health and military institutions across provinces did not exchange vital information. Such fragmented authority was also manifested in Beijing where both the military and civilian systems appeared to suffer from miscommunication at the early stage of the crisis.

However, Lai also suggests that despite all these weaknesses, China's political system is still capable of mobilizing resources to cope with the SARS crisis. The Chinese national authority centralized the administrative control of cadres by penalizing inefficient officials and authorized provincial party and administrative leaders to mobilize various branches of provincial bureaucratic agencies to fight SARS. Apart from allowing localities and institutions to mobilize the resources to combat SARS, central leaders also took the lead in enforcing and coordinating SARS management among bureaucratic agencies, provinces and between Hong Kong and Chinese provinces. While SARS was effectively contained eventually, Lai points out that a lack of formal coordinating authority within the provinces may still exist and such serious drawbacks need to be overcome by the state in order to better cope with any future major crisis.

In his paper, Zou explores how the SARS crisis affected China's ongoing legal reform towards the rule of law. Zou observed that the outbreak of SARS forced the Chinese leadership to consider the important role of the law in realizing good governance. The state was prompted to enact new regulations on public health emergencies which aim to establish a prompt and effective emergency response mechanism to combat SARS. These regulations contain "rule of law" elements such as responsible reporting system, public participation and the punishment of delinquent officials.

Zou found that the poor legal system helped the spread of SARS. The old law was inadequate in its enforcement during the anti-SARS campaign. The law, for instance, did not have any clear provision on whether a hospital has the right to refuse admission of certain patients afflicted with infectious diseases. There was also no provision on legal liability imposed on patients who refused to be quarantined. Moreover, China's low legal consciousness and weak law enforcement also contributed to China paying a "high price" in the fight against SARS. The slow construction of health law and weak law enforcement has nevertheless taught China to respect the law and how to effectively enforce the law. Fortunately, the SARS crisis has made the Chinese leadership realize the importance of a sound legal system.

Gu Xin focuses his attention to China's healthcare system, which bore the brunt of the SARS onslaught, and he tries to show how the inadequacies of China's public health had delayed measures to cope with the crisis effectively. The inadequacies manifested themselves in several aspects. The lack of a universal medical insurance coverage caused those who are uninsured (mostly peasant workers and unemployed urban residents) to delay seeking prompt medical treatment. Furthermore, the commercialization of healthcare providers had resulted in rapid growth of healthcare service costs and as a result, many patients who do not have the financial means simply delay seeking medical attention until their sickness becomes severe. In addition, there is a sharp decline in the state's financing role in both the public and private healthcare services. Consequently, a wide range of public health services are being underprovided.

A more direct link between China's ailing public health system and the SARS crisis lies in the poor mechanism of information dissemination. As observed by other contributors in this volume, Gu also found that the problem of poor information dissemination within the healthcare sector was compounded due to the separation of the military and the civilian healthcare provision. For instance, during the early stages of the SARS epidemic, one of the major reasons for the Beijing municipal government's ignorance of the accurate number of SARS cases was that the army hospitals did not and were not obliged to report their cases to the local authorities.

Beyond public healthcare, Cao Cong reveals serious weaknesses in China's scientific and medical community in responding to emerging new infectious diseases such as SARS. According to Cao, Chinese scientists could have turned the SARS crisis into an opportunity to demonstrate their growing scientific prowess if they had acted together. Unfortunately, China's rigid science and technology management system was partly to blame for having not responded to the crisis quickly and effectively. In the pre-reform era, Chinese scientists from different jurisdictions were able to cooperate on important government-initiated projects and successfully executed them. But since the mid-1980s when China began to reform its science and technology management system, competing interests and rivalry among different scientific research institutes have ensued. The scientific community was incapable of taking initiatives or even coordinating their activities across different jurisdictions since each institution, regardless of its capability and expertise, wants to conduct SARS-related research on its own.

Moreover, even though Chinese scientists and physicians may have done first-rated work in research and patient treatment in fighting against SARS, they were unable to participate and make a contribution to the international pool of scientific knowledge by getting their research published in a timely fashion. The failure to communicate their research findings further exposed one of the important weaknesses of China's science and technology management system.

In addition, the persistent funding constraints meant that not enough resources were committed to the research of SARS. In China, there were doubts whether the research on SARS warrants funding to a level that may not commensurate with the seriousness of the disease. Since other fatal diseases like cancer or AIDS have claimed more lives than SARS, diverting resources to researching SARS implies the negligence of more urgent illnesses.

In his paper, He Baogang discusses how information control impeded China from taking effective measures fighting SARS. From the beginning, the Chinese government was accused of controlling, hiding, distorting and even manipulating information on the SARS virus and the extent of the outbreak. Like other contributors to this volume, He highlighted several reasons to explain the reluctance of the government to release information about the SARS. First, the nature of the authoritarian system of government discouraged officials to reveal information, particularly negative news, which could result in a severe backlash against the state and threaten the legitimacy of the ruling party. Second, the covering up of information was crucial in ensuring social stability particularly during a sensitive leadership transition period which saw Hu Jintao and Wen Jiabao taking over the helm of the party and government within a span of a few months. Third, the Guangdong government was preoccupied with the performance of the local economy and downplayed any negative news. Fourth, the bifurcation of the authority between the civilian and military authorities impeded efforts to curb the SARS outbreak in its initial stages.

SARS IN HONG KONG

In their paper, Thomson and Yow explain how Hong Kong coped with the SARS crisis by looking at the role played by the government and civil society. They found that apart from the measures introduced by the Hong Kong government, the response of the Civil Society Organizations (CSOs) and the general public was crucial in halting the spread of SARS and reducing the fear, confusion and near hysteria at every level of society.

To curb the spread of SARS, the Hong Kong government introduced a number of measures such as instituting screening procedures at immigration checkpoints, closing of schools, introducing quarantine measures and improving healthcare procedures. However, the government also committed a number of mistakes such as its delay in informing the public of the gravity of the situation, its indecision over the closure of the schools and failure to institute timely and adequate quarantine measures.

Even before the SARS outbreak, the people of Hong Kong were already quite disillusioned with the government because of the economic recession and high structural unemployment. When SARS broke out, the people accused the government of its slow and weak responses. Frustrated by the ineffectiveness of the government, the CSOs began to collaborate closely with the former. More than 1,000 CSOs were found to have played a pivotal role in reducing the adverse impact of SARS.

Lessons from the SARS Crisis

A final question can be posed: what have the two governments learnt from the SARS crisis in terms of establishing a sound governance system? During the SARS crisis, most criticisms were targeted at China due to its authoritarian political system. Nevertheless, we believe that every system can learn from such an unprecedented crisis, which has exposed the many "cracks" in the existing system. Specifically, the SARS crisis did lay bare the weaknesses of China's authoritarian system, but it also showed its strengths. Some of our contributors have objectively pointed out that every system has its own advantages and shortcomings. Apparently, both political systems have room for further improvement in order to be effective in coping with sudden social crises like SARS.

Nevertheless, learning is a long process, and the process from the time the lesson is learnt to policy changes is even longer. Our contributors have found that all the relevant segments of society in both China and Hong Kong have more or less learned something from the SARS crisis. But then some policy practices are easier to be changed than others. For instance, any structural change would generally take a longer time than a procedural change.

Would the SARS crisis speed up China's progress towards democratization? In their paper, Zheng and Lye provided an assessment of the impact of the SARS crisis on China's political system. They observed that in the short to medium term, the Chinese leadership is likely to continue with on-going efforts at improving the transparency and accountability of the political system, streamlining the bureaucracy and devising a more comprehensive social security and healthcare system. However, it would be unrealistic and perhaps politically naïve to conclude that the SARS crisis would lead to China's political democratization.

In the same vein, Zou argues that the application of the relevant laws and regulations has helped China win the anti-SARS battle. In this sense, one can hope that China will put more emphasis on the importance of law in future. But it is also unrealistic to expect that this crisis will transform China's legal system. Similarly, Cao shows that there are difficulties in introducing fundamental changes in China's scientific community. Despite being "defeated" by SARS, as Chinese scientists have recognized, existing problematic practices within the community are likely to continue and the scientific community and the leadership have yet to learn their lessons from the SARS crisis and take concrete measures to improve the co-ordination of China's research systems.

In some areas, the Chinese government has already taken serious measures to enhance institutional capacities to cope with crises like SARS. Gu found that as the ailing healthcare system could not effectively handle the SARS crisis, the government has begun to undertake some long-term measures to restructure its public health system in particular and the entire healthcare regime in general. Investment in public health is expected to increase, a national SARS information feedback and dissemination system has since been set up. More importantly, the healthcare system would be strengthened in the rural areas. The government has learned a bitter lesson not to underestimate the importance of investing in such crucial social infrastructure as the healthcare sector if it were to respond promptly to any viral outbreak in future.

For Hong Kong, the most important lesson that the government has learned is that civil society can play an important role in coping with crises like SARS. Thomson and Yow observed that while SARS may have accentuated the problems of the Hong Kong government, it brought the people of civil society together. It helped fostered a sense of solidarity and forced the CSOs, more than ever, to learn to cooperate, possibly creating new political structures for moving out of the increasing intractable political malaise that the territory had been encountering since Hong Kong's return to China.

Chapter 1

The Impact of SARS on Greater China Economies

JOHN WONG, SARAH CHAN AND LIANG RUOBING

OVERVIEW

The recent SARS outbreak struck the Greater China economies as primarily a random and unforeseen event. The impact operates like a cyclical factor, disrupting economic growth through both the demand and supply sides in the short run. The demand shock to the economy is reflected by a fall in consumption. From the supply side, SARS disrupts production and business operations. This will adversely affect both the services and manufacturing sectors. Delays in international shipments of inputs and final commodities may also be experienced as trade is hampered, aggravating the supply-side shocks.[1] The negative external shock of SARS also manifests itself even faster through the financial markets. If the SARS outbreak cannot be effectively contained, fear of the disease may continue to grow, weakening market confidence and depressing stock prices. The wealth effect of these could further aggravate the demand-side shocks.

The external shock arising from the SARS outbreak therefore impacts the Greater China economies very much like a business cycle. Once SARS had subsided, particularly if the epidemic had not been prolonged, the economy could bounce back to growth. Apart from the "cyclical effects", SARS also exposes or perpetuates the structural weak-

[1] "Economic impacts of the SARS outbreak on East Asia: An initial assessment", *Asia Economic Monitor*, at http://aric.adb.org/infocus/sars/spotlight_sars_outbreak.asp.

nesses of the economies, for instance the high structural unemployment, budget deficits and persistent deflation.

Just as significantly, combating the outbreak of SARS entails substantial fiscal costs, including increased expenditures for upgrading medical capabilities and financial assistance to cushion the economic fallout of the outbreak.[2] Increases in fiscal spending may come along with declines in revenue mobilization as economic growth slows. The diversion of government expenditures away from investments in public services, which are growth-enhancing and have higher multiplier effects, to SARS-related expenditures also implies economic costs. The fiscal implication will be most significant for Hong Kong where its fiscal position is already weak compared to its neighbors like China and Taiwan.

Nonetheless, the strong economic fundamentals of the Greater China economies should help them to weather external shocks. China, Hong Kong and Taiwan has been able to withstand the fallout from SARS in varying degrees. For China, SARS has not dented its economic growth; prior to the outbreak of the deadly epidemic, China was already expanding nearly 10% year-on-year in the first quarter and after SARS, the economy registered a sharp recovery by growing 9.1% in the third quarter after plunging 6.7% in the second quarter as a result of the viral outbreak. For Taiwan whose economy was already slowing down before the SARS crisis, the effects of SARS appear to be short-lived as the economy bounced back to respectable growth, underpinned by a moderate recovery in exports and industrial production. Hong Kong was the worst hit compared to China and Taiwan. SARS dealt a double whammy to its economy which was already mired in recession before the crisis occurred. Lost revenue from tourism further compounded the weak local consumption expenditure and exacerbated the already worsening unemployment situation. Even when SARS was brought under control, economic recovery at best remained weak, incipient and fragile as Hong Kong continued to be plagued by persistent deflation, serious structural unemployment and high budget deficit.

CHINA

The Chinese economy has been steaming ahead with strong growth before the outbreak of SARS. Whereas the 1997 Asian financial crisis

[2] *Ibid.*

brought down many regional countries, the Chinese economy was hardly affected by the turmoil as it continued to grow at 8.8% in 1997 and 7.8% in 1998. After the crisis, while economic growth in most of Asia had fallen to low or negative rates (Figure 1) and the global economy at large was creeping into recession, China's economy alone was still steaming ahead with strong growth, chalking up 7.3% growth for 2001 and 8% for 2002 (Figure 2). Recently, China has shown that its economy after SARS could bounce back to growth much faster and stronger than other Asian economies which were brought down by such an external shock.

The recent SARS outbreak in fact exerted only a temporary and short-term effect on the Chinese economy. After a rapid 9.9% growth in the first three months of the year, economic growth slackened and grew a modest 6.7% year-on-year in the second quarter (Figure 3). After SARS, the economy expanded 9.1% in the third quarter compared to the same period last year. Due to the strong rebound and the potentially faster rate of growth in the fourth quarter, GDP growth for 2003 is officially estimated by the National Bureau of Statistics to reach 8.5%.

Manufacturing, which accounts for half of all economic output, initially suffered the effects of the epidemic. As seen from Figure 4, the impact of SARS is more evident in April and May, where the industrial output growth was clearly lower than the 17% increase in March. However, the fallout from SARS remained limited. In June, industrial output surged by a strong 17% to US$363 billion as various sectors rebounded after the SARS outbreak. In November, the month for which the latest data is available, industrial output rose 17.9% on a year-on-year basis.

On the trade front, China's economy is already starting to shrug off the impact of SARS. China's exports posted robust growth of around 30% in the four consecutive months of April, May, June and July (Figure 5). The SARS outbreak has a lagged impact on exports in August, with exports growing at a slower pace than July even though it grew 27% compared to the same period a year ago. In September, exports picked up and surged by more than 31% from a year earlier. In the first three quarters, exports and imports totaled US$308 billion and US$299 billion, up

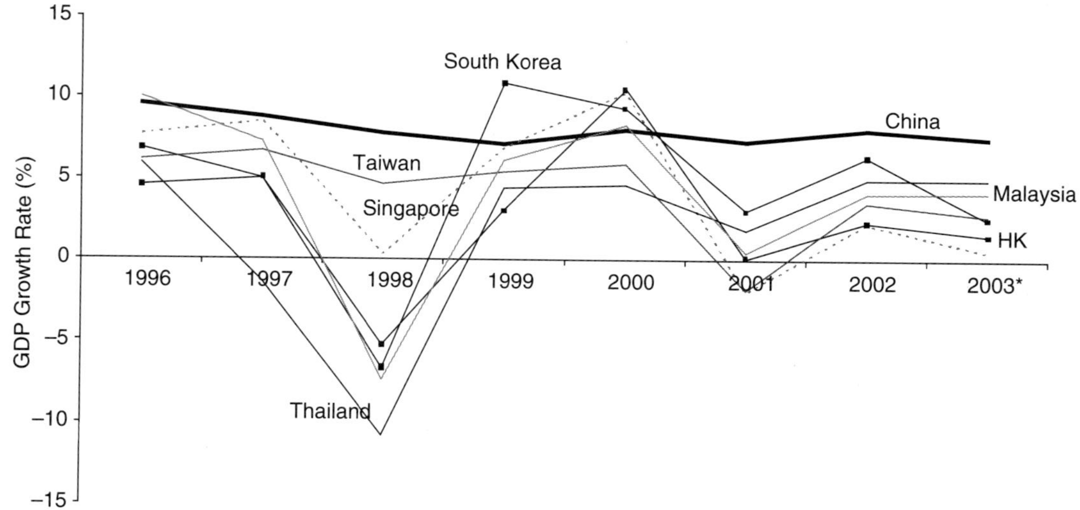

Figure 1. Economic Performance of China and the Asian Economies, 1996–2003*

*2003 growth forecast estimated by IMF in its World Economic Outlook, September 2003.

Sources: World Bank, "East Asia regional update: Making progress in uncertain times", 6 Nov 2002; Asian Development Outlook 2002.

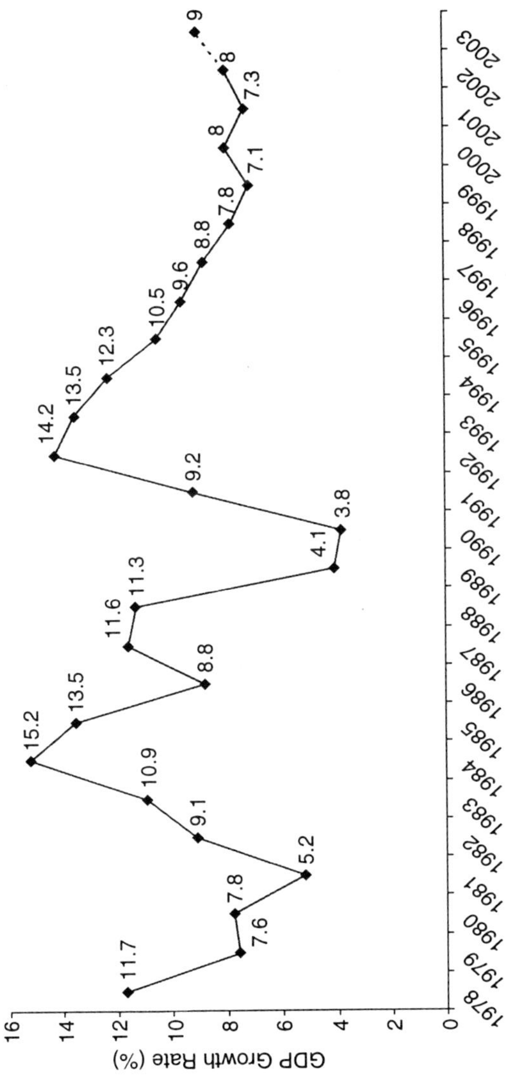

Figure 2. China's Economic Growth, 1978–2003*

*Denotes estimate.

Sources: *China Statistical Yearbook*, various editions.

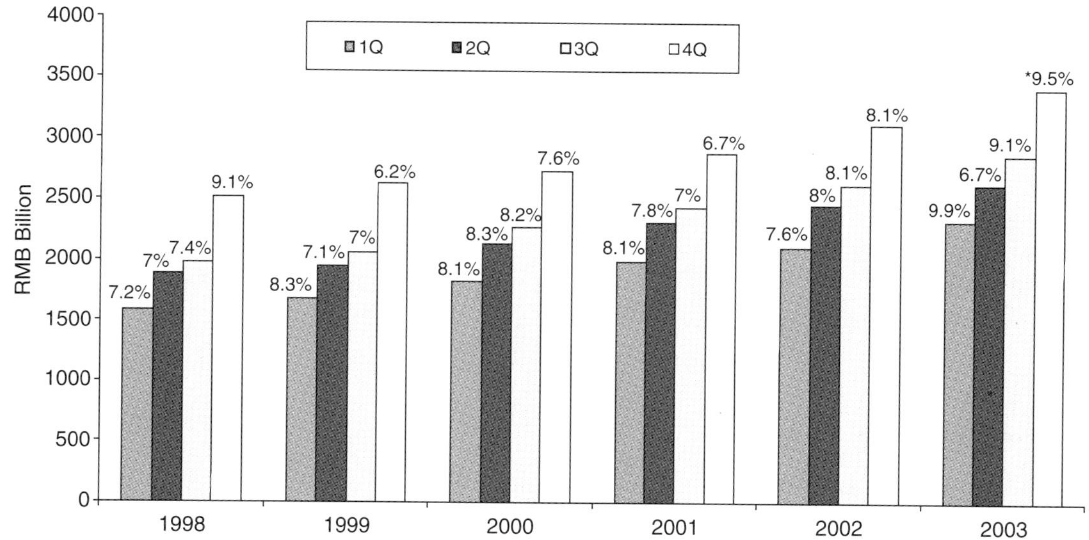

Figure 3. China's Quarterly Growth Rate, 1998–2003*

*The level of quarter GDP is in current price and the quarter growth rate is calculated in constant price.

Sources: The People's Bank of China, *Quarterly Statistical Bulletin*, various issues; *China Monthly Economic Indicators*, Oct 2002 issue.

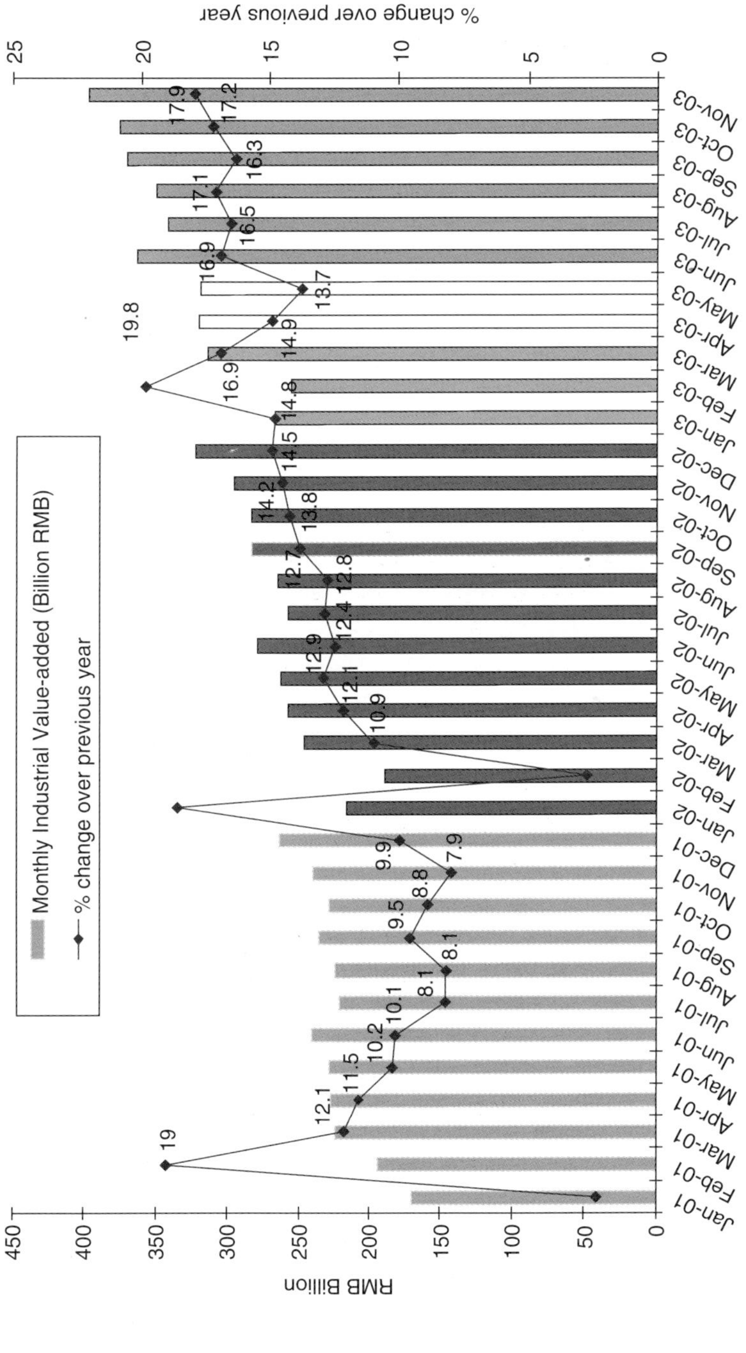

Figure 4. China's Industrial Production, 2000–2003*

*Denotes latest data available at time of writing.

Source: *China Monthly Statistics*, various issues.

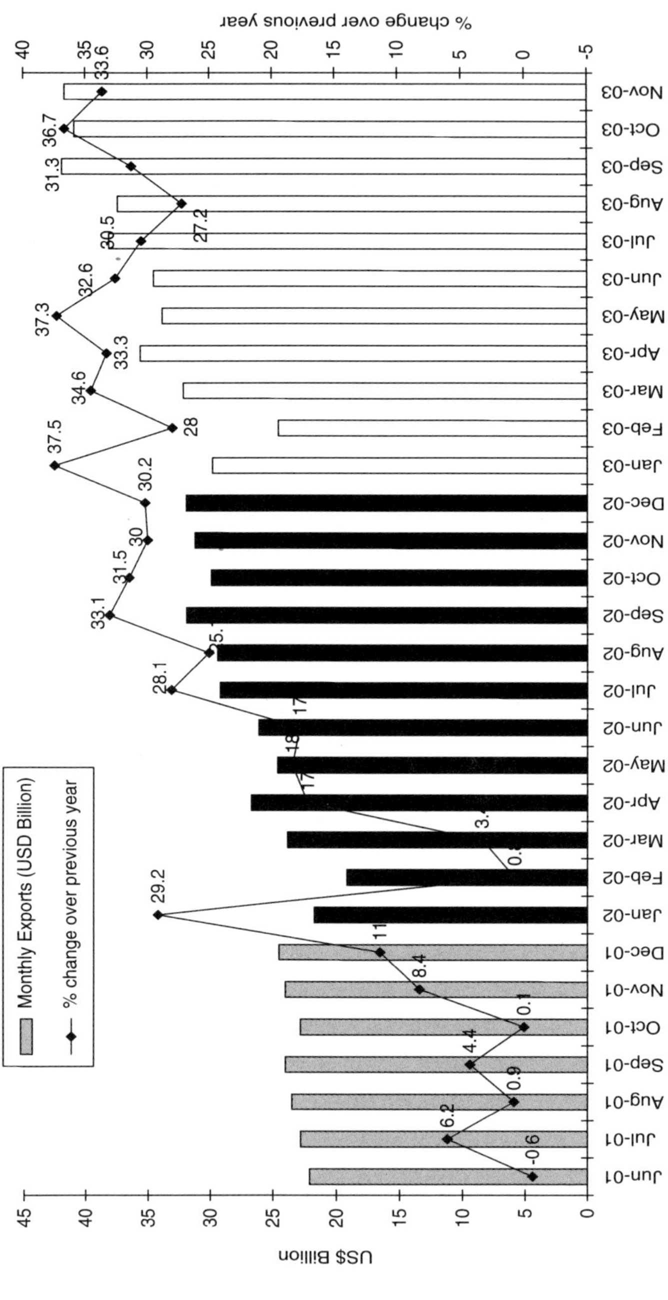

Figure 5. China's Exports, 2001–2003

Source: Data from Ministry of Commerce, http://www.mofcom.gov.cn.

32.3% and 40.5% respectively.[3] The latest trade figures suggest China's economy is emerging relatively unscathed from SARS.

SARS has not undermined the fundamentals of the Chinese economy. It may have heightened investors' perception of risk in China but for most firms, the risks continued to be outweighed by attractions of China's high productivity, low labor cost and huge domestic market. At the peak of the SARS epidemic in May this year, for instance, foreign direct investment (FDI) increased by almost two-fifths to reach US$5.5 billion (Figure 6). FDI also rose by 12% in the first nine months of this year to reach US$40 billion. Despite SARS, FDI in China is estimated to total about US$57 billion, US$4.3 billion more than that in 2002.

The initial economic impact of SARS is felt on the services sectors. Revenues in the services sectors — retail, tourism, hospitality and entertainment industries — have dwindled. In April, revenue from the food and beverage sector plunged by as much as 50%, however sectors like pharmaceuticals and healthcare goods (like body fitness equipment) enjoyed brisk sales. The insurance sector seemed to be immune; insurers' premium in Beijing rose 38.4% year-on-year in April. In other cities like Guangdong and Shanxi, it rose 17.1% and 82.5% respectively.

SARS threw the tourism and transportation sector into a tailspin. In Beijing, tourist arrivals plummeted by nearly 60% in April from a year earlier. In May, civilian passenger volume reportedly dropped a drastic 78% compared to the same period a year ago. Domestic tourism was almost virtually at a standstill for the whole month of May. At the end of June, about 70% of domestic airline capacity had been restored but the seat occupancy has averaged less than 50%. Due to the strong battering of SARS, international airlines were adversely affected in June; passenger volume to China were only 25–30% of last year preceding period's level. The Chinese media have estimated the travel industry lost about US$33 billion during the SARS crisis.[4]

As a result of the negative impact on the services sectors which is particularly vulnerable to consumer confidence and spending, the

[3] "China reports 36.2% rise in foreign trade", *China Daily*, 17 Oct 2003.

[4] "China break boost travel", *China E News Alert*, No. 35, Oct 2003.

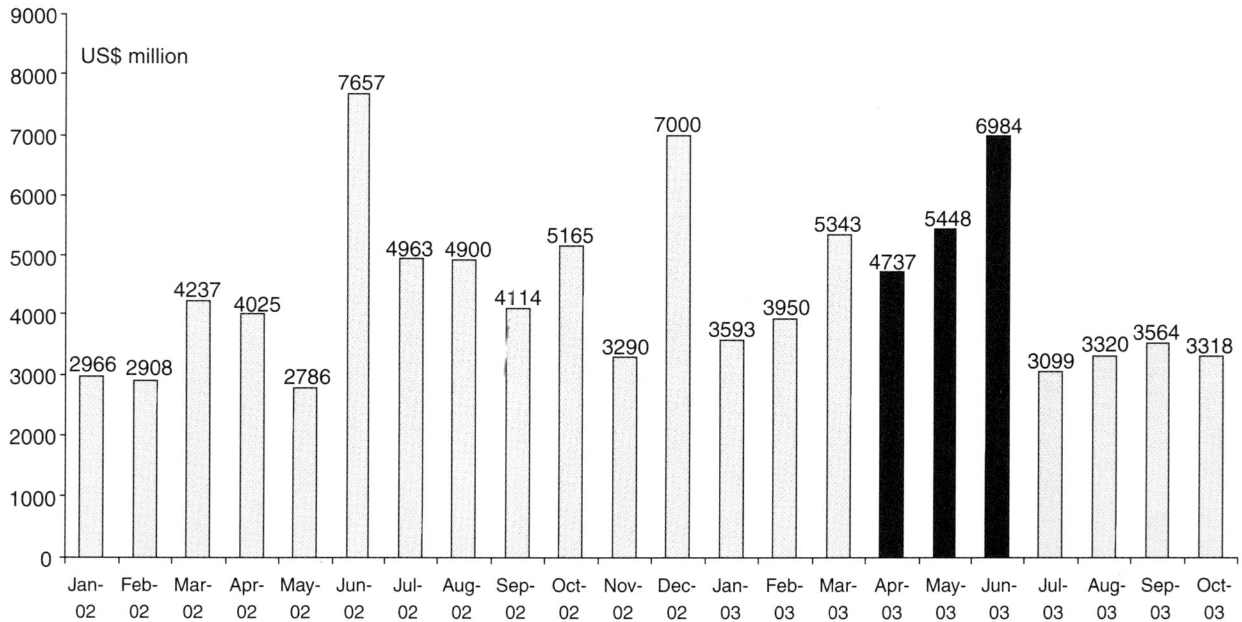

Figure 6. China's FDI, 2002–2003*

*Denotes latest data available at time of writing.

services industry in China grew only 0.8% in the second quarter, a drop of 6.1 percentage points compared with that of the same period last year. However, in the third quarter, recovery in the services sector has evidently resumed, with an increase of 7.6% year-on-year.[5]

SARS also exerted a negative impact on retail sales, due to a weakening in demand from consumption. Retail sales in April rose 7.7% over a year ago, compared to an increase of 9.3% year-on-year in March (Figure 7). Overall sales for the whole month of May were depressed by an extremely weak restaurant sector and the cancellation of the Golden Week holiday in early May. However, this was offset by sales of medicines, automobiles and as a result, retail sales rose a moderate 4.3% year-on-year in May. Consumer sentiment however appeared to quickly recover from SARS. As SARS is contained and triggered a revival in shopping, retail sales in June grew 8.3% from a year earlier, double the pace at the height of SARS epidemic in May. In July, retail sales rose 9.8%, suggesting that consumer spending had rebounded. It expanded at a slower rate in September, at 9.5% compared to a year ago.

As a result of the SARS epidemic which contributed to slow economic activity, consumer prices rose a mere 0.3% year-on-year in June, compared to the previous month which rose 0.7% year-on-year (Figure 8). Reflecting weakening demand for commodities, retail prices declined by 0.6% in May from a year ago, which was a sharp drop of 0.7 percentage points compared to April. As the economy recovers from SARS, overall consumer prices grew 0.5% and 0.9% respectively in July and August. In September, China reported a 1.1% rise from a year earlier in consumer prices, contributing to a 0.7% increase in the first nine months of 2003.[6]

The SARS crisis further aggravated the serious unemployment situation in China. According to a recent report in the Chinese Academy of Social Sciences, the outbreak deprived 8% of rural workers of their jobs in the urban areas.[7] The labor market is estimated to lose 1.3 million jobs this year due to SARS. The spread of SARS exacerbated difficulties for

[5] "Sars impact to GDP growth estimated 0.8%", *Xinhua*, 17 Oct 2003.

[6] "China's economy not 'overheated': NBS official", *China Daily*, 18 Oct 2003.

[7] "Economists call for efforts to combat SARS-caused unemployment", *China Daily*, 2 Jul 2003.

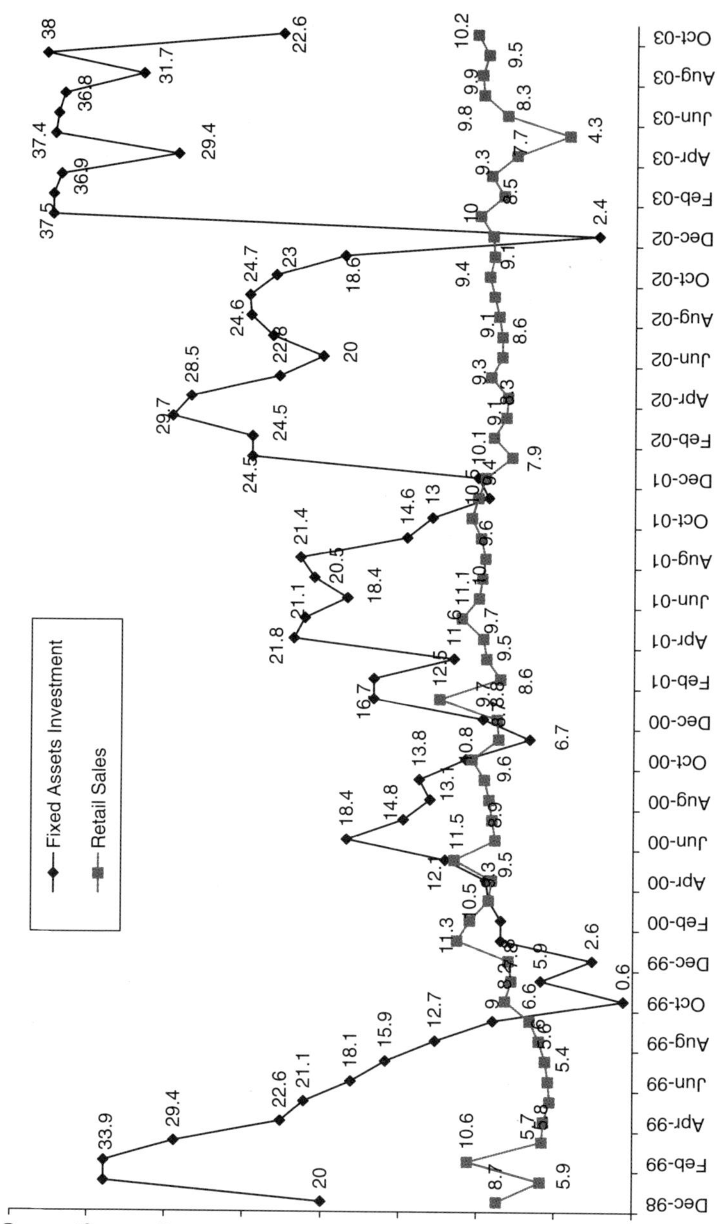

Figure 7. China's Domestic Consumption and Investment, 1998–2003*

*Denotes latest data available at time of writing.

Source: China Monthly Statistics, various issues.

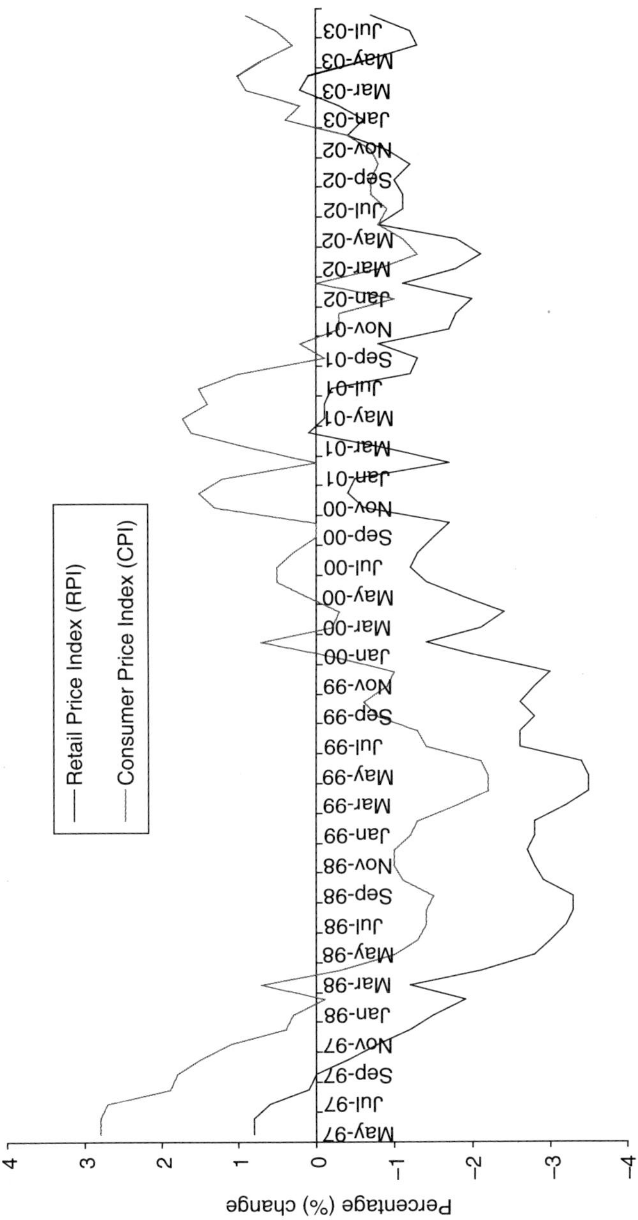

Figure 8. Deflationary Pressures in China, 1997–2003*

*Denotes latest data available at time of writing.

Source: The People's Bank of China, *Quarterly Statistical Bulletin*, various issues; *China Monthly Statistics*, various issues.

China to create new jobs; it is estimated that the official unemployment rate will hit 4.5% in 2003, 0.5 percentage point more than that of 2002.[8]

To insulate the economy from the worse effects of the SARS, the government increasingly relies on capital investment to pump-prime the economy. In January–September 2003, fixed asset investment grew by 31% year-on-year.[9] The surge in investment growth has been driven by an acceleration in money supply growth. Broad money, or M2, has grown by more than 20% year-on-year in recent months,[10] as seen from Figure 9. Partly due to China's strong external economic balances, i.e., current account surplus, FDI influx and speculative inflows in anticipation of RMB revaluation, the pick-up in money supply growth is also attributed to a rapid growth in loans which in turn fuel over-investment in capacity. In the first eight months of the year, Chinese financial institutions extended loans totaling 2.1 trillion yuan, double the amount over the corresponding period last year.[11]

The acceleration in M2 growth has triggered concerns that there could be downward pressure on already soft prices but at the moment, inflationary pressures remain weak. Some sectors however appear to be overheating. In 2000–2002, for instance, property or real estate investment grew by more than 22% year-on-year; in the first eight months of 2003, the rate of growth accelerated further, to 33% year-on-year.[12] Other sectors like steel, nonferrous metals and building materials are also at risk from over-investment. Due to the increased demand for automobiles, investment in the iron and steel industry grew by a phenomenal 130% in the first six months of 2003.[13]

To cool the overheating economy, the People's Bank of China (PBOC) on 21 September 2003 moved to raise the bank reserve ratio by one percentage point (from 6% to 7%) to tighten credit and reduce excess liquidity of around US$18 billion in the banking system.[14] It also

[8] *Ibid.*

[9] "Fixed asset investment in China up 22.6% in October", *The Business Times*, 18 Nov 2003.

[10] Loans in the first half of 2003 exceeded the total granted in all of 2002. See "Is China's boom in danger", *BusinessWeek*, 3 Nov 2003.

[11] "Central bank moves to treat economy's Achilles' heel", *The Straits Times*, 20 Oct 2003.

[12] "Is China's boom in danger", *Business Week*, 3 Nov 2003.

[13] *Ibid.*

[14] *Ibid.*

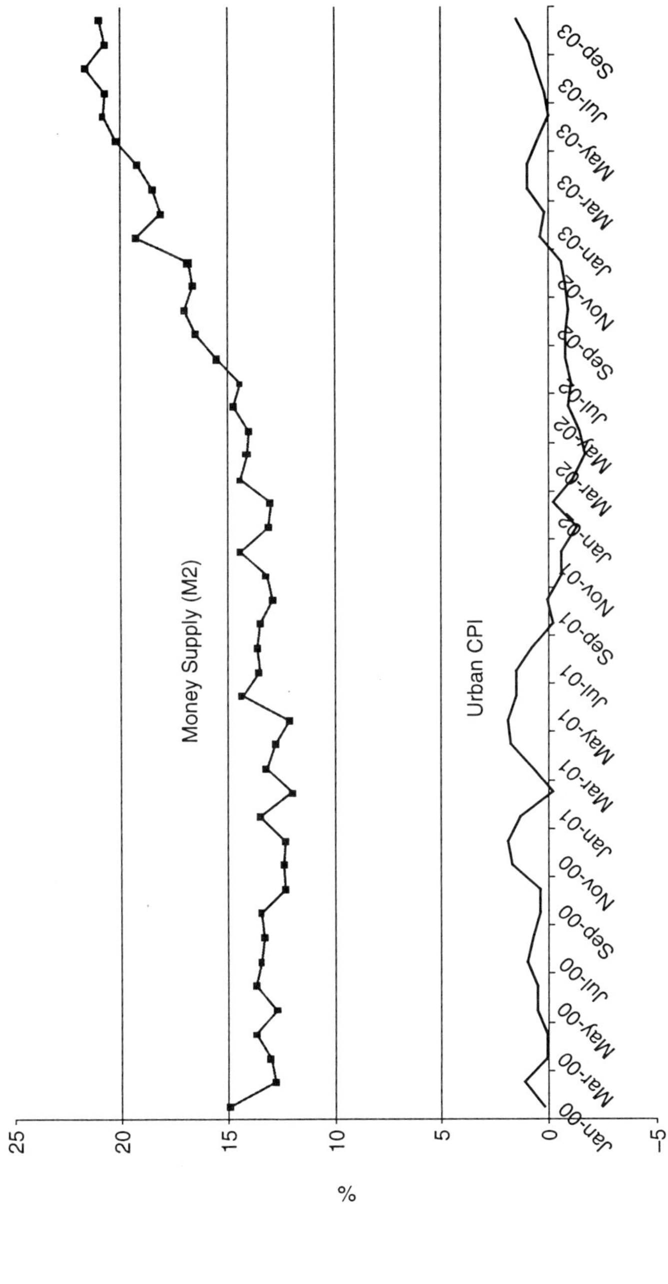

Figure 9. Money Supply and Prices, 2000–Date

Source: China Monthly Statistics, various issues.

passed a directive on June 13 to tightened regulations on lending to the property sector, stipulating that developers will not be eligible for bank loans unless they put up at least 30% of the project cost out of their own pockets.[15] However, it is uncertain if such monetary policy measures will prevent overheating of the Chinese economy without stalling economic growth. If the latest measures fail to check investment growth, the central bank may pursue more aggressive action by raising interest rates. The economy may be geared for a hard landing if that happens.

TAIWAN

Taiwan's economy was already slowing down before SARS due to the US recession and global slump in electronics exports. The SARS-induced downturn however proved short-lived for Taiwan's economy and most of the return to growth was cyclical. In the first quarter of 2003, the economy continued to grow at a rate of 3.5% but contracted by 0.1% in the second quarter due to the outbreak of SARS (Figure 10). It grew 4.2% year-on-year in the third quarter and is estimated to expand 4.7% in the fourth quarter. As the economy steadily recovers from the impact of SARS, the official growth rate is forecasted to be 3.2% for 2003.[16]

The initial impact of SARS is felt on the services sectors. According to a report by the Cabinet's Council of Economic Planning and Development, tourist arrivals to Taiwan in April reportedly fell by 50–60% compared to the same period last year and hotel occupancy dropped by more than 30% (refer to Table 1). Domestic tourism is expected to be badly hit and is estimated to fall by as much as 70% in May as people avoid travelling due to fear of catching SARS. As governments and companies impose travel restrictions to SARS-affected areas, and tourists cancel holiday booking, passenger volume to Taiwan declined by as much as 80% in the first week of May while airline carriers grounded

[15] "Property fund to make its debut", *China Daily*, 11 Aug 2003.

[16] "Taiwan's strong GDP increase spurs Taipei to raise forecast", *Asian Wall Street Journal*, 17 Nov 2003.

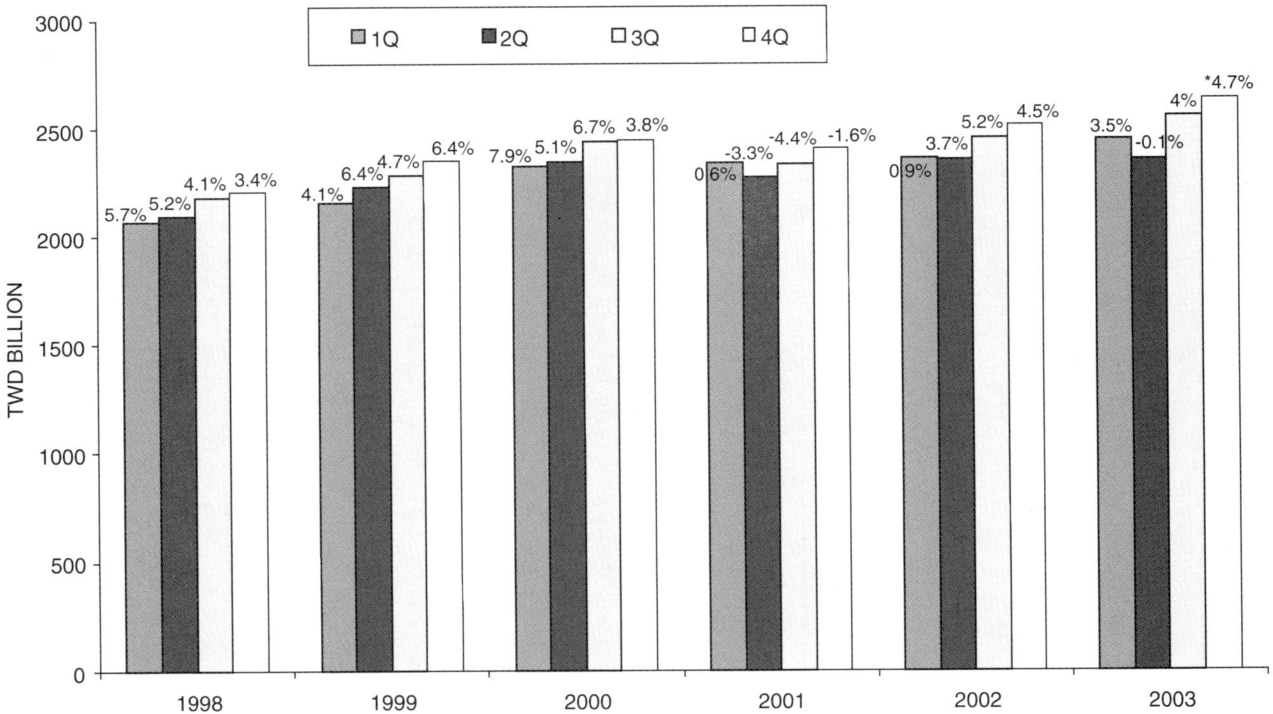

Figure 10. Taiwan's Quarterly Growth Rate, 1998–2003*

*GDP at constant 1996 prices. The Cabinet's Council for Economic Planning and Development officially forecast 4th quarter growth rate to be at 4.7%.

Source: Taiwan Economic Forum.

Table 1. Recent Indicators: Impact on Service Sectors in Taiwan

Sector	March 2003 (yoy % change)	April 2003 (yoy % change)
Tourism		
Outbound tourism (%)	−21.63	−64.53
Tourist arrivals (%)	−0.21	−50.66
Hotel occupancy rate (%)	Decline of 3% or more	Decline of 30% or more
Aviation (flight cancellation, passenger volume)	Cancellation rate of air flights 24%; passenger volume (7 Mar–12 May) decline by 53%	
Media (movie attendance)	−3.76%	−31.5%

Source: Report by Council of Economic Planning and Development, Taiwan, 19 May 2003.

up to 24% of the flights. However, Taiwan's tourism-related services is expected to be the least hit by SARS compared to Hong Kong and China since tourism receipts accounts for only 1.4% of its GDP.

The performance of Taiwan's manufacturing sector has deteriorated sharply since March. As seen from Figure 11, industrial output expanded by just 1.8% in March, and proceeded to contract in both April and May due to SARS. The sector did, however, begin to recover in June when overall production rose by 2.3% year on year. After SARS was brought under control, industrial production improved considerably and rose 7.5% before slowing to 5.3% in August. Industrial output in the eight months to August grew 3.6%.

Taiwan's trade performance experienced a marked slowdown due to the SARS crisis. The slowdown in trade growth was most pronounced in May, which grew 2% compared to the same period in 2002, at a rate lower than April's export growth of 5.5% (Figure 12). Export growth in June remained weak, growing at 3.3% compared to the same period a year earlier. As the seriousness of the outbreak began to ease in June, export growth returned to double-digit territory after July and rose 13% year-on-year in August. In September, export growth hit a moderate 12% despite growing at a slightly slower pace compared to the previous month.

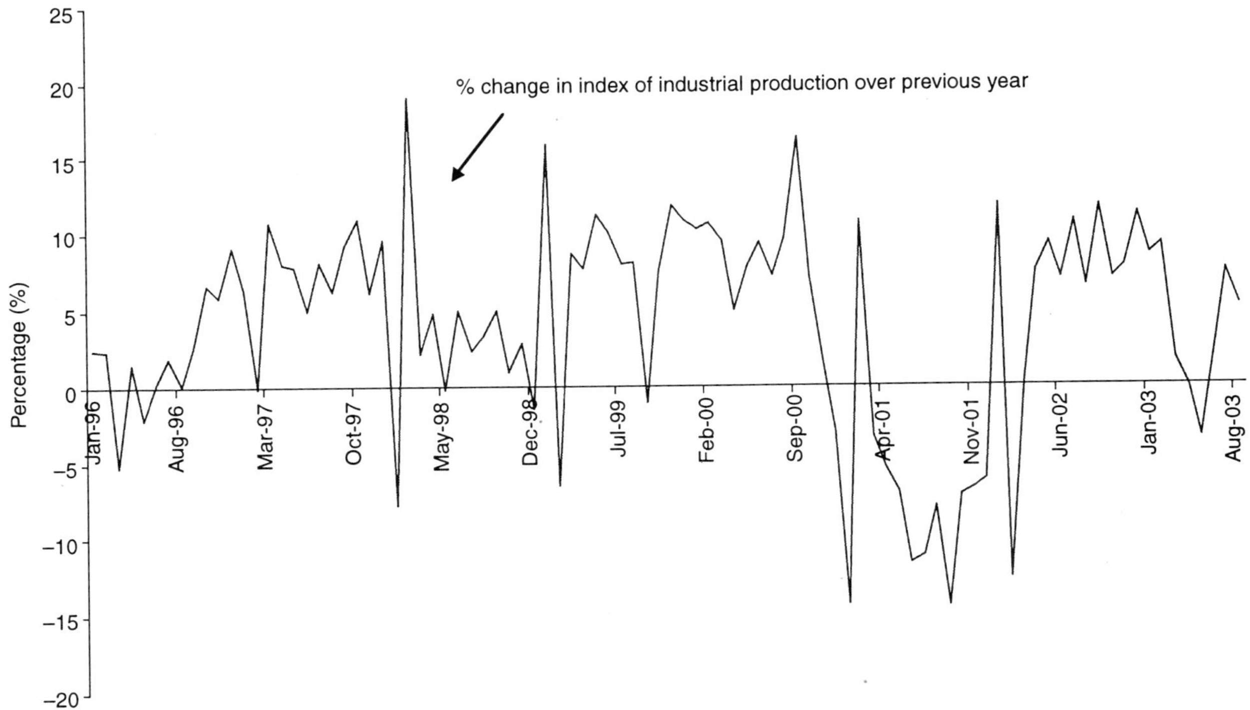

Figure 11. Taiwan's Industrial Production, 1996–2003*

*Denotes latest data available at time of writing.

Sources: Derived from Directorate-General of Budget, Accounting and Statistics, *Monthly Bulletin of Statistics*.

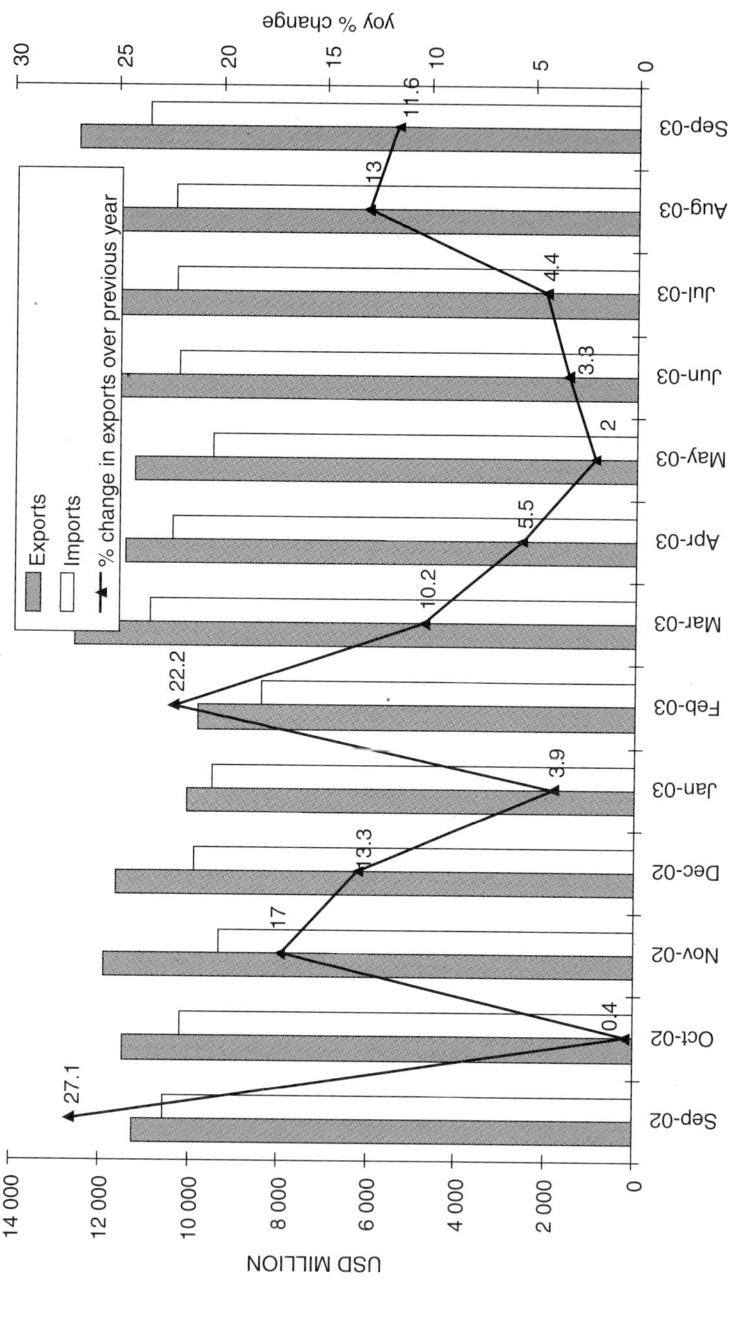

Figure 12. Taiwan's Foreign Trade, September 2002–2003*

*Denotes latest data available at time of writing.

Source: Ministry of Economic Affairs, http://www.moea.gov.tw.

Unemployment in Taiwan rose from 4.9% in April to 5.1% in June, partly due to the SARS outbreak and partly as a result of rising first-time job seekers (Figure 13). According to the Directorate-General of Budget, Accounting and Statistics (DGBAS), the slump in economic activity caused by SARS contributed to a rise in the number of people made unemployed, owing to the closure or downsizing of businesses, from 429,000 in April to 433,000 in May.[17] The non-seasonally adjusted unemployment rate continued to hover above 5% in June but Taiwan's joblessness rate is expected to fall further in the final months of the year as the economic recovery from the SARS crisis gains momentum and two government-funded programs to provide temporary employment opportunities get under way.[18]

Inflation is unlikely to be a problem in Taiwan for some time. The softness of overall consumer prices in Taiwan is nothing new and the SARS crisis further exerted downward pressure on already soft prices. The CPI declined by 0.6% year on year in June, due in part to the SARS outbreak (Figure 14). The fall in prices in the subsequent months of July, August and September continued even after Taiwan was declared a SARS-free area on 5 July and consumption activity started to return to normal. Some structural factors no doubt contribute to the softness of prices. Falling world prices for durable goods such as PCs is one. By increasing competition in the domestic economy, the implementation of market-opening measures that began even before Taiwan entered the WTO in early 2002 is also putting downward pressure on prices in particular sectors of the economy. Prices in Taiwan have also been held down by weak investment demand and an ailing banking system.[19]

Hong Kong

The SARS outbreak could not have come at a worse time for Hong Kong, whose economy was already facing a serious recession with rising unemployment and low growth. As seen from Figure 15, unemployment

[17] "Unemployment rises", *EIU Viewswire*, 25 Aug 2003.

[18] "Unemployment falls to two year lows", *EIU Viewswire*, 22 oct 2003.

[19] "Weak inflationary forces", *EIU Viewswire*, 25 Aug 2003.

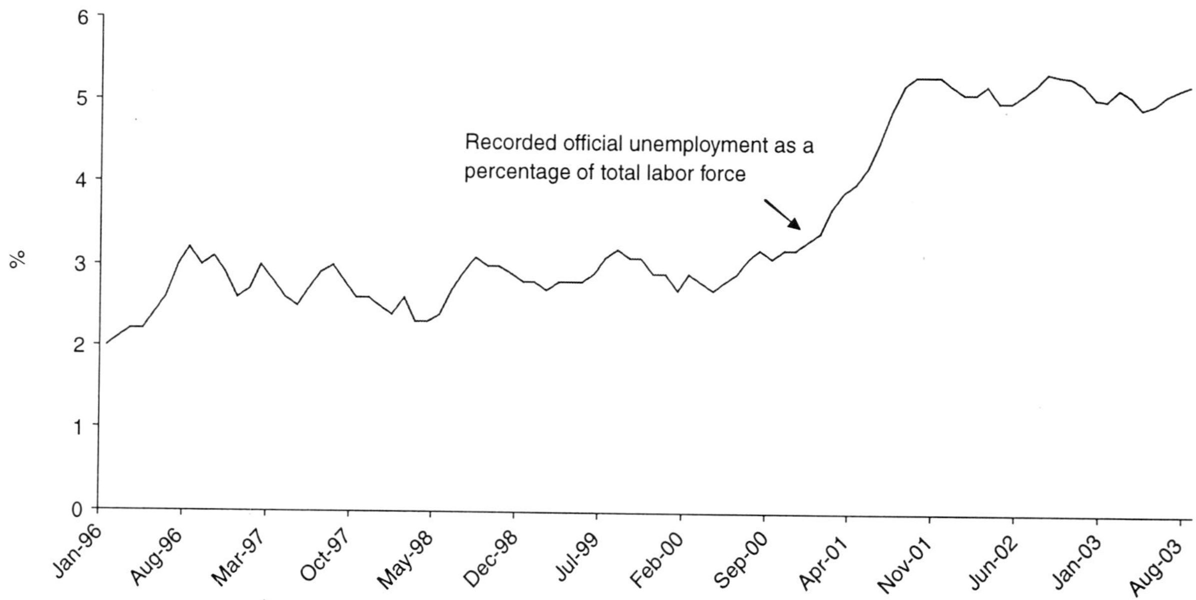

Figure 13. Official Unemployment in Taiwan, 1996–2003*

*Most recent data derived from Directorate-General of Budget, Accounting and Statistics. Non-seasonally adjusted.

Source: Directorate-General of Budget, Accounting and Statistics; Taiwan Statistical Data Book; Taiwan Economic Forum (TEF).

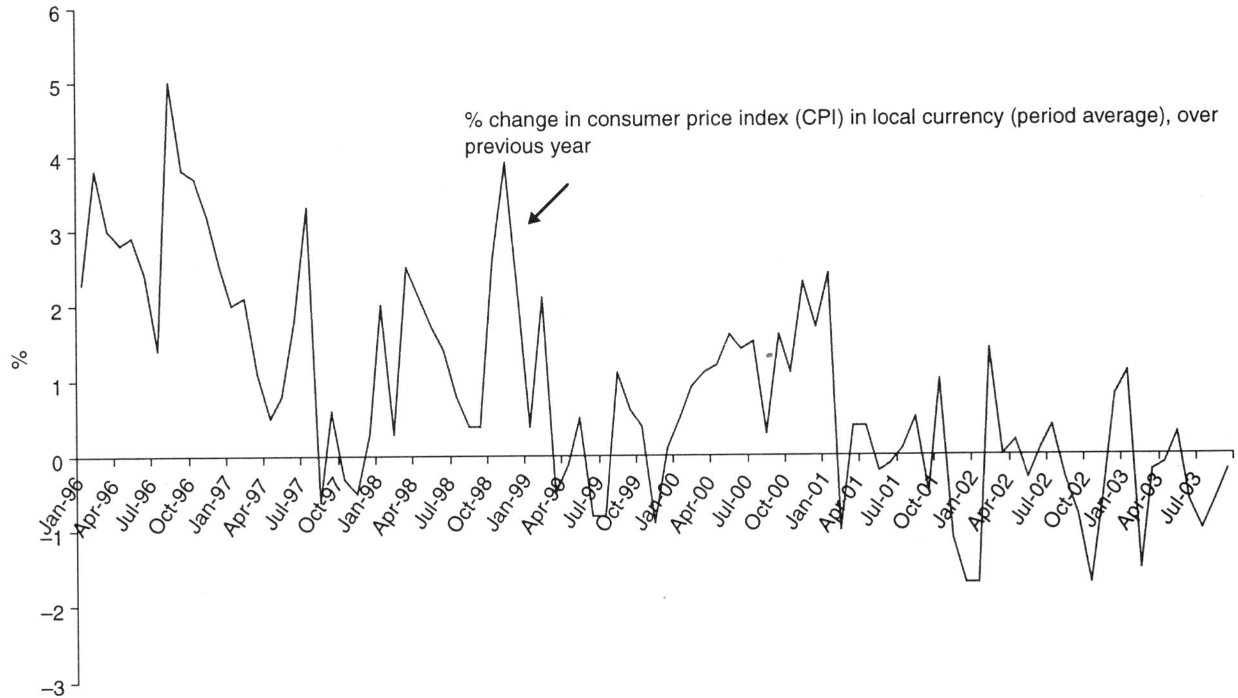

Figure 14. Low Inflation in Taiwan, 1996–2003*

*Denotes latest data available at time of writing.

Source: Derived from Council of Economic Planning and Development.

was at a high of 7.8% in 2002 while economic growth was only 2.3% in the same year. With the spread of SARS in mid-March 2003, Hong Kong's economic woes were further exacerbated. In the second quarter of 2003, real GDP contracted by 0.5%, down from an increase of 4.5% in the first quarter (Figure 16). Economic growth rebounded in the third quarter and grew 4% from a year earlier,[20] as consumption witnessed a pickup due to a rise in PRC tourists as a result of relaxed travel rules for Guangdong residents. Recent government forecast for 2003 is estimated to be at 3% (from the previous forecast of 2%), the second revision in two months to reflect the rapid recovery from SARS.

Among the Greater China economies, HK's tourism-related services including airlines, hotels, restaurants, entertainment and retail trade, was the worst hit by SARS since tourism receipts account for 5.1% of its GDP (Figure 17). Tourism indicators have headed south since the SARS outbreak started. International passenger traffic was reportedly down by 50% since mid-March, with many flights scheduled for April being cancelled. Hong Kong Airport Authority reported an 80% drop in passenger numbers at its Chek Lap Kok airport in May.[21]

For inbound tourism, the total number of tourists coming to Hong Kong rose by 19.7% in the first quarter of 2003. However, the SARS outbreak dragged down the number by 57.9% in the second quarter. There have been signs of improvements since then. The drop in the number of tourist arrivals moderated to 5.6% in July, before returning to an increase of 9.6% in August. For the first eight months as a whole, the number of tourist arrivals dropped by 14.4% from the same period a year earlier. Effective from January 2002, the quota system for mainland tourists under the Hong Kong Group Tour Scheme was abolished. Accordingly, the number of mainland tourists travelling to HK soared by 18.6% in the first eight months of 2003, despite a fall of 26% in the arrivals of mainland tourists in the second quarter amid the SARS fallout. Mainland residents from Beijing, Shanghai, Guangzhou, Shenzhen, Zhuhai, Zhongshan,

[20] HK's GDP rose by a seasonally adjusted 6.4% from the second quarter. "Post-Sars HK rebounds with 6.4% growth", *The Straits Times*, 29 Nov 2003.

[21] "Economic impact of the Sars outbreak on East Asia: An initial assessment", *Asia Economic Monitor*, at http://aric.adb.org/infocus/sars/spotlight_sars_outbreak.asp.

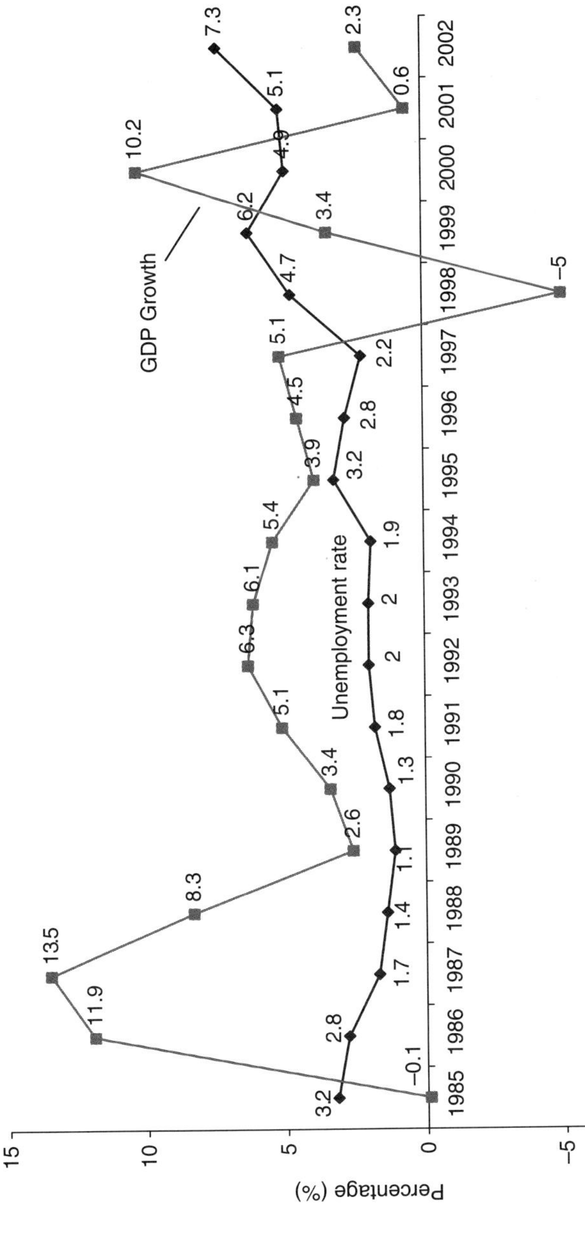

Figure 15. Growth and Unemployment in Hong Kong, 1985–2002

Source: HKSAR Census and Statistics Department.

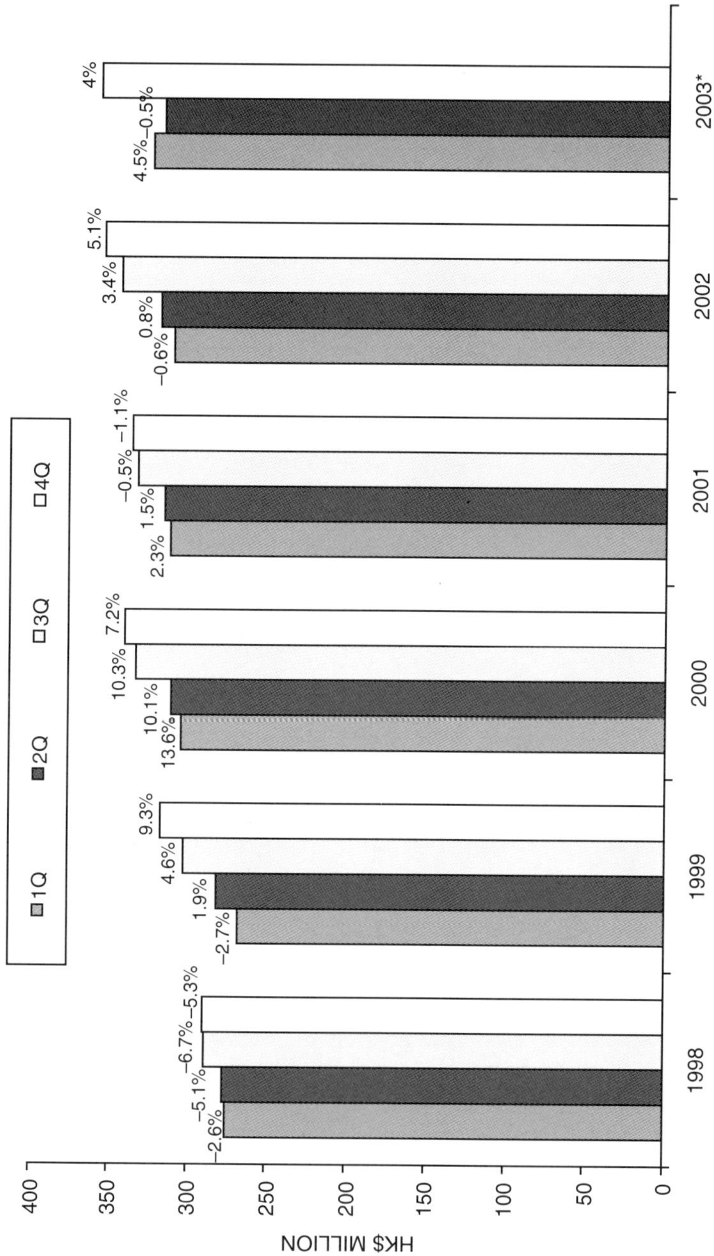

Figure 16. Hong-Kong's Quarterly Growth Rate, 1998–2003*

*Percentage change is in real GDP, over the previous year.

Source: HKSAR Census and Statistics Department.

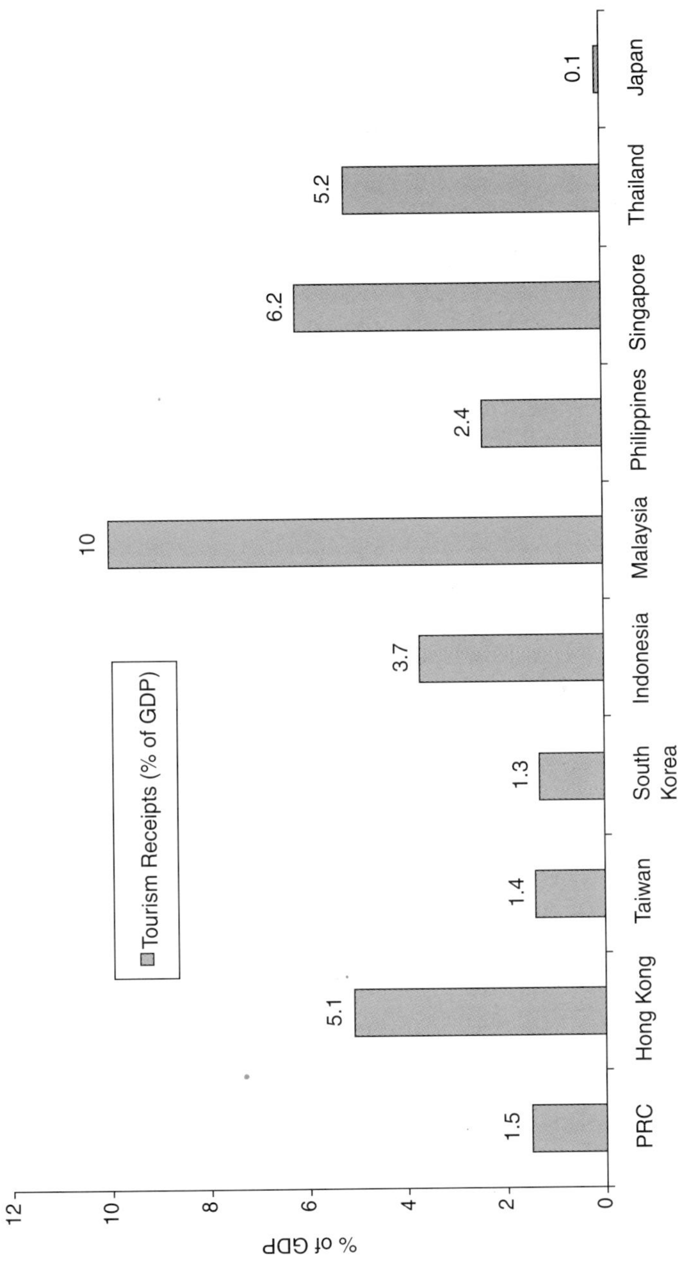

Figure 17. Tourism Receipts, Selected Asian Countries, 2001

Source: Standard & Poor's. "SARS will crimp Asian growth but not sovereign ratings", 22 Apr 2003.

Foshan, Dongguan and Jiangmen are now allowed to travel to Hong Kong as individuals, rather than as part of tour groups. This relaxation scheme has provided a boost to HK's tourism industry.[22]

Domestically, consumer spending remained lacklustre amid the worsening employment condition and the continued weakness in the asset markets. Local sentiment was weak even before the SARS outbreak and as consumers further restrain their spending after the epidemic, retail sales fell by 11.1% in May from a year earlier, after dropping by 15.2% in April. The impact of SARS bottomed out in June as retail sales fell at a slower pace of 3.3%. For the first seven months of 2003, retail sales dropped by 6.2% in value, further slackening from a decline of 4.1% for 2002 as a whole.[23]

Reflecting the generally subdued local demand conditions, falls in overall prices have continued to widen, caused in part by continuing declining property values. The Composite Consumer Price Index (CCPI), which covers 90% of households, has dropped for four consecutive years, by 1.6% in 2001 and 3% in 2002.[24] The SARS crisis further intensified HK's persistent deflationary pressures, causing consumer prices to decline by 4% in July from a year earlier, after dropping 2.5% in May and 3.1% for July (Figure 18). In September, the fall in prices eased slightly amid an economic recovery and growth in tourism, as the CCPI fell 3.2% compared to a year ago. The slower pace of decline was mainly attributable to an influx of visitors from China, which help relieve some of the downward pressure on prices.[25]

Labor market conditions were also weak and have been drained recently by the SARS outbreak. The unemployment rate reportedly surged to a worse-than-expected new record of 8.3% in March–May 2003, as seen from Figure 19. In June, the official unemployment rate was 8.3%, aggravated by SARS and new entrants to the workforce. For the

[22] "Economic & trade information in Hong Kong: Current economic situation", at http://www.tdctrade.com/main/economic.htm#5.

[23] *Ibid.*

[24] *Ibid.*

[25] "Hong Kong index suggests easing in deflation trend", *Asian Wall Street Journal*, 24 Oct 2003.

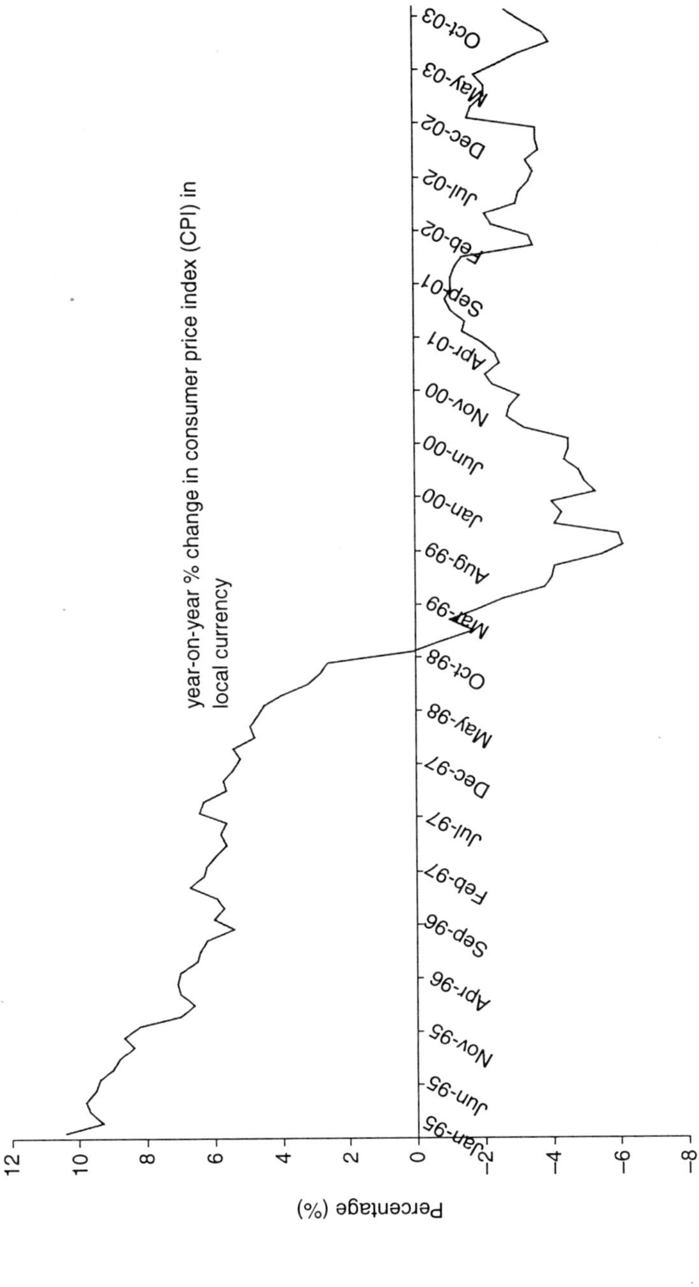

Figure 18. Deflation Trend in Hong Kong, 1995–2003

Source: Hong Kong SAR Government Census and Statistics Department, *Hong Kong Monthly Digest of Statistics*.

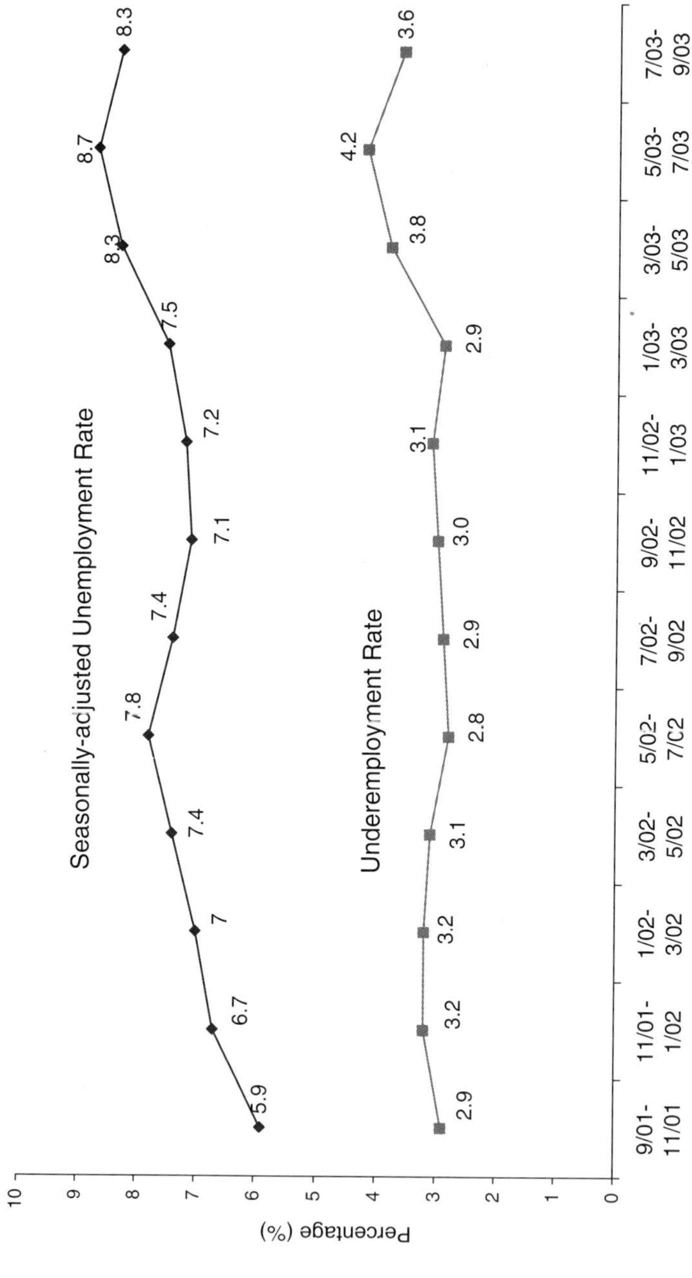

Figure 19. Unemployment and Underemployment in Hong Kong, 2001–Date

Source: HKSAR Census and Statistics Department.

May–July quarter, unemployment was at a record rate of 8.7%, reflecting both the impact of SARS and continued underlying weakness of the economy. The seasonally-adjusted unemployment rate eased and dropped to 8.3% in the three months ended September 2003, while the underemployment rate, which measures the percentage of the labor force that is less than fully employed, fell to 3.6% from 4.2% for May to July, due to an improvement in the overall economy and the influx of mainland tourists from China.[26]

Hong Kong's economic growth for 2003 is expected to see a V-shaped recovery as exports remained resilient with the territory's growing integration with the Pearl River Delta, a weak US dollar and the current US-led global recovery. In April 2003, total merchandise exports only grew by 9% year-on-year partly because of the SARS crisis and partly due to weak sales to the US arising from the Iraq war (Figure 20). As the impact of SARS waned, Hong Kong recorded improved exports in June compared with the same period last year, growing at 14% year-on-year after rising 13.6% in May. Imports rose 11.5% after an increase of 9.4% in May. Exports appear to have emerged from the SARS outbreak unscathed; for the first six months of 2003, the value of total exports rose 14.7% and imports rose 13.4% compared to same period last year. The government attributed HK's strong export resilience to brisk trade in East Asia, particularly the mainland's robust external trade performance.

Hong Kong's index of industrial production registered a decline of nearly 9% in the first quarter of 2003 compared to the same period last year. Due to SARS, the industrial production index further fell by 13% in the second quarter (Figure 21). Reportedly, the manufacturing sector is heading towards a moderate recovery in June. The Purchasing Managers' Index (PMI), an indicator of future manufacturing activity, climbed past the 50 mark which is higher than May's PMI which was 41.2. (Any reading above 50 indicates expansion of manufacturing sector). July PMI posted a reading of 51.4, up slightly from 50.2 in June and staying above the no-change 50-mark for the second straight month. A recovery of business activity is expected in the third quarter.

[26] "Hong Kong posts lower jobless rate", *Asian Wall Street Journal*, 21 Oct 2003.

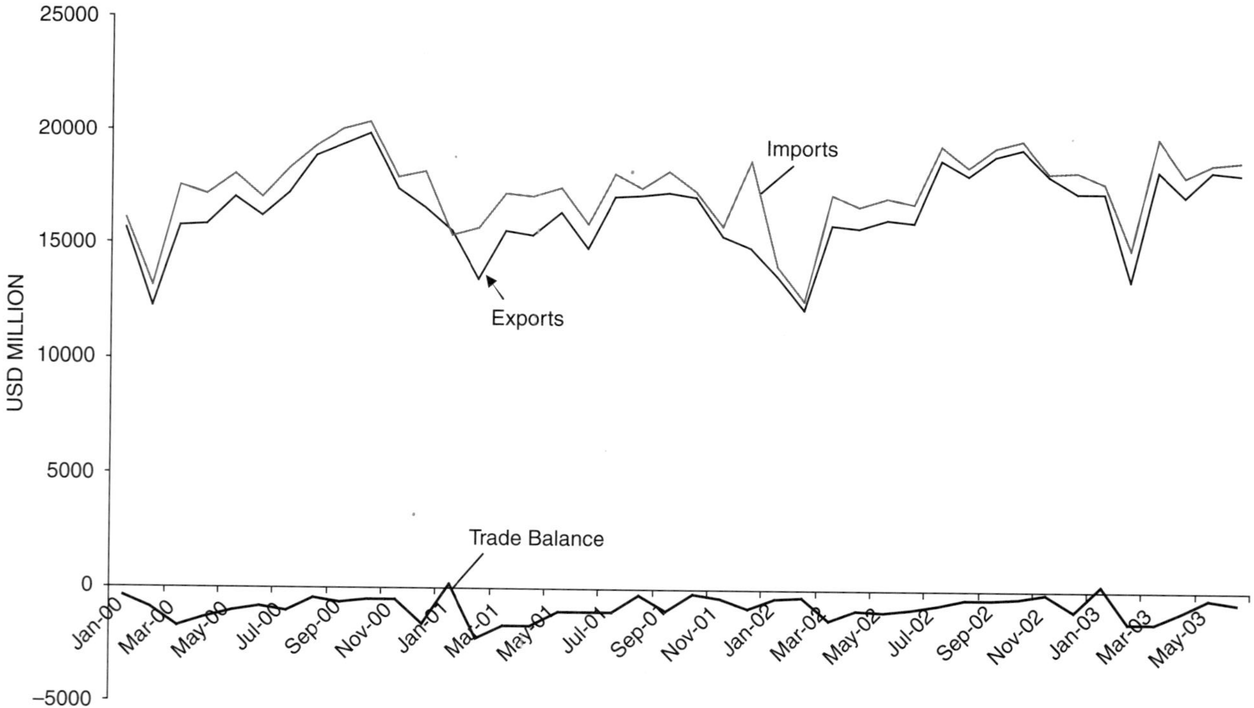

Figure 20. Hong Kong's Aggregate Merchandise Trade Values, 2000–Date

Source: Hong Kong SAR Government Census and Statistics Department, *Hong Kong Monthly Digest of Statistics*.

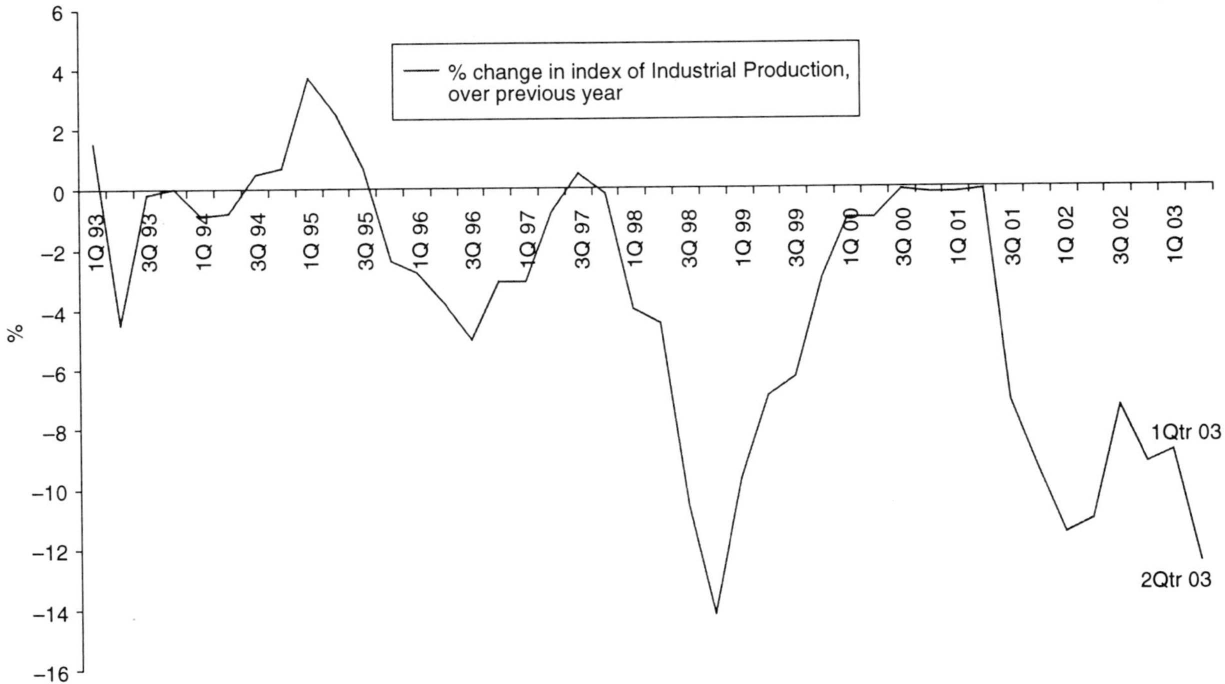

Figure 21. Hong Kong's Industrial Production, 1993–2003*

*Denotes latest data available at time of writing.

Source: Hong Kong SAR Government Census and Statistics Department, *Hong Kong Monthly Digest of Statistics*.

Chapter 2

SARS and China's Political System

ZHENG YONGNIAN AND LYE LIANG FOOK

The outbreak of the severe acute respiratory syndrome (SARS) and efforts to contain it have posed what is generally regarded as the first major political test to the Hu Jintao–Wen Jiabao leadership since they took over the helm of the party and government. The coronavirus that supposedly originated from the small municipality of Foshan in Guandong Province soon spread uncontrollably to other provinces in China and even abroad. The political fallout from its tenacious spread took the leadership by surprise and showed up weaknesses in China's political system.

Like other countries, crisis management provides an interesting angle for scholars to examine the weaknesses and strengths of a given political system. This also applies to China. Traditionally, quite a number of scholarly literature on China was generated by crises occurring in the country such as the great famine followed by the Great Leap Forward and the Cultural Revolution in the Mao Zedong era, and the 1989 pro-democracy movement and 1999 Falun Gong movement since Deng Xiaoping's reform and open-door policy.

The SARS outbreak has again turned the spotlight on China's political system. An examination of how this system has handled the SARS outbreak will not only give us an idea of how the regime has faired in the midst of the challenges posed by the new environment, i.e., globalization, market economy and social mobility, but also some sense of the direction the Chinese political system is likely to head.

This paper is divided into five sections. The first section seeks to contextualize China's initial poor and delayed response to the SARS outbreak. The second section examines the weaknesses of China's political system from four dimensions, i.e., bureaucratic fragmentation, central-local relations, civilian-military relations, and urban-rural divide. As a balance, the third section discusses the strengths of China's political system in coping with SARS. The fourth section looks at how China's leaders, namely Hu Jintao and Wen Jiabao have responded to pressure generated from outside the country, and finally, the fifth section attempts to spell out the political implications of SARS.

CONTEXTUALIZATION OF THE SARS OUTBREAK

It is worth highlighting at the outset that SARS is a new form of atypical pneumonia and it took a while for China as well as other governments to recognize its tenaciousness.[1] Scholars have compared how different governments have responded to the SARS outbreak and why some governments,

[1] A report prepared by the World Health Organization has said, "SARS needs to be regarded as a particularly serious threat for several reasons. The disease has no vaccine and no treatment, forcing health authorities to resort to control tools dating back to the earliest days of empirical microbiolog: isolation and quarantine. The virus comes from a family notorious for its frequent mutations, raising important questions about the future evolution of outbreaks and prospects for vaccine development. Epidemiology and pathogenesis are poorly understood. The initial symptoms are non-specific and common. All available diagnostic tests have important implications. If tests are poorly conducted or results wrongly applied, patients excreting virus and thus capable of infecting others can slip through the safety net of isolation and infection control. The disease continues to show a disturbing concentration in previously healthy hospital staff — the human resource vital to control. A significant proportion of patients require intensive care, thus adding to the considerable strain on hospital and healthcare systems. Evidence is mounting that certain source cases make a special contribution to rapid spread of infection. The maximum incubation period, currently estimated at ten days, allows spread via air travel between any two cities in the world. WHO's most recent analysis estimates overall case fatality in the range of 14% to 15%. In persons over the age of 65, the case fatality ratio can exceed 50%." See report entitled "Severe acute respiratory syndrome (SARS): Status of the outbreak and lessons for the immediate future" dated 20 May 2003, prepared by World Health Organization Communicable Disease Surveillance and Response.

e.g., Singapore, have performed better than others, e.g., Taiwan government. To some extent, this reflects the nature of governance in different countries. But before we explore how China's governance affected its response to SARS, we have to first understand the political context in which the outbreak took place.

There are three major characteristics of China's political context, namely political priority, political correctness, and non-transparency. Each of them will be looked at in detail below, particularly their impact on China's response to SARS.

One distinctive feature of China's political context is that there is usually no clear distinction between matters that belong to the political realm and those that lie outside of it. In many democratic countries, whether a particular event becomes political or not is often the result of the confluence of several factors such as public opinion, public pressure, positions taken by politicians and the role of NGOs and interest groups. This is because the public forms an essential component of the political process through its access to various avenues of political participation. Hence, when a social event occurs, the public can immediately make known its views and even influence the course of events.

In China, the public's participation in the political process is less straightforward and not necessary guaranteed. Whether an event comes under the political realm or not is more often than not shaped by the perceptions and actions of top leaders, either collectively or individually. Not everything is regarded as having a political significance, and not every issue is resolved politically. There have been occasions where a particular issue, even when it is serious, is handled by local governments or central bureaucracies, and top leaders choose not to get involved. In other instances, the public may take matters into their own hands by engaging in demonstrations or public protests although such actions clearly fall outside the realm of permissible behavior. Even then, the central government may decide not to intervene and leave it to the local authorities to handle. It is usually after a social event is deemed to have entered the realm of politics and assumes a political significance that top leaders begin to pay attention to it.

This was what happened to Falun Gong. Initially, Falun Gong was regarded as a "useful" organization that helped to fill a social gap in

China's spiritual vacuum. Falun Gong had been active in parts of China for many years, and in some locations its followers even had brief skirmishes with public security forces. But the public security agencies did not care to report such "small matters" to the top leadership. In 1997, Falun Gong followers protested against the Beijing city government in front of Beijing TV station. Although this incident became well known locally, the top leader paid scant attention to it. It was only until Falun Gong grabbed international headlines by "laying siege" to Zhongnanhai (the communist leadership compound) in 1999 did the top leadership regard it as a serious threat to the existing social and political order. Its attitude to the movement hardened overnight. Over the next few years, the regime mobilized every available means to crush the movement.[2]

The manner in which the SARS outbreak was handled bears some resemblance to the above. When the first two SARS cases were found in Guangdong in November 2002, the patients were diagnosed then as having "un-identifiable" pneumonia. Although the early spread of SARS did cause some panic, neither Guangdong nor Beijing perceived the matter seriously. In February and early March 2003 when SARS spread to different parts of Guangdong and Hong Kong, it was still regarded as a medical issue, not a political one. Hence, the matter should be handled by local governments, and at most by relevant central bureaucracies such as the Ministry of Health. At that time, although those who were infected began to die, SARS had not yet entered the realm of China's politics. Only when SARS went beyond China and reached Taiwan, Singapore, Canada and other parts of the world and resulted in mounting international pressure did the top leadership somewhat belatedly begin to regard SARS as political issue and started to mobilize national resources to combat its spread.

A second major characteristic of China's political context which partly explains the Chinese government poor and delayed response to

[2] China's top leaders reacted in a similar harsh manner to the activities of China's Democratic Party in 1998 which they perceived as a direct challenge to the authority of the Chinese Communist Party (CCP). Over a few months of that year, the preparatory committees of China's Democracy Party were established in twenty-three out of China's thirty one provinces and major cities. Furthermore, applications to register the new party were made in fourteen provinces and cities. This was unacceptable to the CCP and the China Democratic Party movement was crushed.

SARS is the prevalent culture of being "politically correct". This essentially means that all party and government organizations as well as related organizations should constantly bear in mind the big picture (为大局着想) and not behave in a manner that would jeopardize the interest of the party or government. Such an approach would include managing the flow of information that would cast the regime in the best possible light. To be sure, the practice of political correctness is not only unique to China but also prevalent elsewhere. The difference between China and elsewhere is often a matter of degree.

In China in particular, a conventional political practice is that good things can and should be exaggerated, but bad things should not receive publicity or should even be hushed up if possible. During Mao Zedong's era, party ideology served as an effective tool to inform party cadres and government officials what they should talk about and what they should avoid. Following Deng Xiaoping's reform and open-door policy, the leadership has become more technocratic and pragmatic, and ideological orthodoxy as a guide to behavior has become less important. Nevertheless, "never report a bad thing during seasons of high politics" has become a norm and is part of the mind-set of Chinese party cadres and government officials.

One of the key reasons why SARS was able to spread from China to other countries was because the local media was not allowed to report on it and as a result, other foreign governments were not forewarned and could not put up safeguard measures in time to stop its import. As mentioned above, the first cases of atypical pneumonia emerged in Guangdong in November 2002 but it was only in February 2003, almost three months later, that the WHO received a report from the Chinese Ministry of Health of an outbreak of a typical pneumonia said to have affected 305 persons and caused five deaths in Guangdong.[3] In early April 2003, a WHO team was finally granted permission to visit the province and was only then able to confirm that the cases that have emerged in Guangdong were consistent with the definition of SARS. SARS had by

[3] SARS was first identified in Vietnam on 28 Feb 2003 when Dr. Carlo Urbani, an epidemiologist from the WHO office in Hanoi, examined a patient with a severe form of pneumonia with no known cause. Source: WHO website at www.sars.int. See also "Officials act as fears over virus outbreak spread", *South China Morning Post*, 12 Feb 2003.

then spread to Hong Kong, Vietnam, Singapore, Toronto and other provinces in China.

When atypical pneumonia was first sighted in Guangdong, several local newspapers did publish some articles on it, but a media gag was subsequently imposed and several journalists were criticized and even removed. Why did this happen? Among many factors, the most important was that the period from October 2002 to March 2003 was the high season of China's politics. In October, the Chinese Communist Party (CCP) held its 16th Congress, the most important event once every five years, which saw the fourth generation leaders led by Hu Jintao taking over the helm of the party. Then in March 2003, China held its 10th National People's Congress (NPC) during which a new government under Premier Wen Jiabao was formed.[4]

In the run-up, during and immediately after these two important events in China's political scene, the emphasis was on creating a "conducive" environment, e.g., maintaining nationwide stability and ensuring minimal disruption to preparations for these two events. Prior to the party congress, the party's propaganda machinery went into overdrive extolling the achievements of the party and calling on cadres to rally together in the interest of the party.[5] After the party congress, another wave of media blitz highlighted the party's formal adoption of the "three represents" theory and it being the "vanguard of the Chinese people and Chinese nation". Likewise, before and after the 10th NPC in March 2003, the official newspapers provided much coverage to issues such as

[4] Zheng Yongnian, "Feidian yu zhongguo zhengzhibing" (SARS and China's political sickness), *Yingxiang fengbao* (Singapore: World Scientific Publishing, 2003), pp. 4–17.

[5] Party discipline was tightened in the run-up to the 16th Party Congress. Wu Bangguo, for one, exhorted cadres not to start or spread political rumors or say anything to tarnish the image of the Party or country. He also called on cadres not to publicly contradict the policies or strategies decided by the Party but to channel their opinions internally. See "Kaichuang guoyou qiye dangjian gongzuo xinjumian" (Opening a new chapter in party building within the State-Owned Enterprises), *Qiushi*, 16 Apr 2002. Luo Gan separately called on the Party and government to be vigilant against disruptive elements such as terrorism, ethnic separatism, religious extremism, internal and external threats, and the Falun Gong movement. See "Zhongyang yanfang wulei puohuai shili" (Party Central heightens vigilance against five types of destructive forces), *Ming Bao*, 10 Apr 2002.

sustaining economic growth, creating employment, lessening the burden on peasants and increasing their incomes.[6] No newspapers were allowed to disseminate any information on SARS during these few months so as to avoid triggering public panic.

In March 2003, some deputies to the National People's Congress had pressed the relevant authorities on why they could not be more forthcoming about the SARS situation in the country. Huang Xirong, a Guangdong People's Congress delegate from Chaozhou had asked the Guangdong Health Department why they did not make a public announcement about such a serious disease earlier. The reply from the local health authorities was that they were afraid of the impact of the disease on tourism and investment because they did not know how to treat the illness.[7] In early April 2003, in a highly unusual move, all 36 Hong Kong deputies to the National People's Congress jointly wrote a letter to NPC Chairman Wu Bangguo urging him to order mainland health officials to release information about atypical pneumonia outbreaks.[8] Hong Kong was by that time reeling from the onslaught of the SARS outbreak.

A third major characteristic of China's political context which has contributed to the leadership's poor and delayed response to SARS is the lack of accountability in the political system.[9] Traditionally, when a

[6] "More economic opportunities expected in 2003", *China Daily*, 12 Dec 2002. See also "Conference backs Zhu's economic strategy", *South China Morning Post*, 11 Dec 2002.

[7] "Province hushed up disease to protect economy, says lawmaker", *South China Morning Post*, 30 Mar 2003.

[8] "NPC deputies call on the mainland to release details", *South China Morning Post*, 2 Apr 2003. See also "HK politicians urge mainland to share their knowledge", *South China Morning Post*, 29 Mar 2003.

[9] Although China's political system is not a representative democracy and its leaders not popularly elected, this does not necessarily mean that the system is not responsive to the needs of its people. To continue to stay in power, the top leadership in the Party and government are acutely aware of the need to stay relevant and be in touch with the aspirations of the people. The development of a market economy has tied the legitimacy of the leadership to its ability to deliver economic goods. In other words, there is an implicit social contract between the regime and its people although the nature of this social contract has changed from upholding communist orthodoxy to producing economic goods. Inherent in this contract is the possibility that if the government fails to keep to its side of the bargain, the people could resort to non-constitutional means to show their displeasure.

mishap or disaster occurs in any part of the country, the *modus operandi* of the government is to try to isolate the affected area and control the dissemination of information to other non-affected areas. The idea is to keep from as many people as possible any bad news so as to minimise any potential political fall-out to the regime.[10] Such an approach was made all the more possible previously when travels by its citizens within and without the country were restricted and less frequent. In this way, a serious matter can be reduced in scale whereas a small matter reduced to nothing (大事化小，小事化无). However, this approach has become less applicable. In an age of globalization and rapid advances in technology, its people travel more often and is more well-informed.

On the SARS outbreak, one of the early assumptions held by Guangdong authorities and even those higher up was that it was necessary to keep a tight lid on news on the outbreak of the disease to prevent mass panic from causing social disorder. Maintaining social stability was to be the guiding principle that should dictate the government's response to the disease. To be sure, initial news that SARS was spreading to different parts of Guangdong in February 2003 did spark off a wave of panic buying by local citizens of essential items such rice, salt and oil.[11] Guangdong health officials were then forced to provide public assurance that the situation was under control when actually it was not.[12] The prevalent thinking then was that it was preferable to work behind the scenes to bring SARS under control. If this was successful, then SARS would not become an issue and life would quickly return to normal. Such a thinking did not preclude officials from painting a false picture of the seriousness of the disease to its own public. To a large extent, the lack of accountability of the political system made this possible. At that time, the leadership did not see the need to respond to outside pressure (both domestic and international) unless the matter becomes a political issue.

[10] "China's response to illness illustrates tradition of keeping disaster hidden", *Associated Press*, 28 Mar 2003. See also "Dictatorships and disease", *International Herald Tribune*, 18 Apr 2003.

[11] "Guangdong moves to curtail panic buying", *South China Morning Post*, 14 Feb 2003. See also "Rumors spark the great salt rush", *South China Morning Post*, 14 Feb 2003 and "Killer bug causes panic in Guangdong", *Straits Times*, 12 Feb 2003.

[12] "Outbreak is now under control, say officials", *South China Morning Post*, 13 Feb 2003.

Weaknesses of China's Political System

The dismissal of Minister of Health Zhang Wenkang and Beijing Mayor Meng Xuenong marked a major turning point in the Chinese government response to the SARS outbreak. By that time, SARS was no longer regarded as merely a medical problem to be resolved by the local governments as they deemed appropriate but had become a political issue that called for a concerted national response. It took a while for this change of perception to occur. Why did the central government not get into the act earlier to contain the outbreak? There are several reasons for this delayed response each of which will be examined below.

The first reason has to do with the economic and political dynamics of Guangdong. As mentioned, local newspapers in Guangdong did initially carry reports on the SARS outbreak. But why did the Guangdong provincial government decide to impose a media gag? There were political and economic actions behind its actions. From the economic perspective, Guangdong, being the biggest trading province in China, is highly dependent on foreign investments and tourism (from Hong Kong and Macao). The concern of local officials was that news of SARS would result in chaos and social instability and thus affect the flow of investments and tourists into the province. This would have a significant impact on its economic performance.

At the political level, Guangdong was experiencing a local power transition from late 2002 to early 2003. In November 2002, Party Secretary Li Changchun was appointed a member of the Standing Committee of the Political Bureau in Beijing. It was clear then that Li would soon vacate his post in Guangdong. Within the same month, Zhang Dejiang, previously Party Secretary of Zhejiang, was appointed to take over Li's position in Guangdong.[13] In January 2003, deputy governor and former Guangzhou Party Secretary Huang Huahua was promoted to become governor of Guangdong. Both Zhang and Huang were appointed largely because of their proven economic track record deemed essential to

[13] "New provincial CPC chiefs appointed in Shandong and Guangdong", *Xinhua News Agency*, 23 Nov 2002.

contribute to the economic vibrancy of the Pearl River Delta region.[14] Thus the top priority of these two leaders was to sustain Guangdong's high economic growth. Even when Zhang Guangning was elected mayor of Guangzhou in late March 2003, he did not comment on the outbreak of atypical pneumonia in Guangzhou in his maiden speech. Instead, he vowed to build on the efforts of his predecessor and achieve higher growth goals.[15] Given the local leadership's preoccupation with Guangdong's economic performance, any news that could affect such a performance such as the SARS outbreak was most unwelcome. Thus, local reports about SARS were suppressed. Hence, not only the central government but also the public in Guangdong was not able to get enough information on this new virus.

Second, the peculiarity of central-local relations also contributed to the spread of SARS. There was a strong inclination on the part of the Guangdong authorities in the initial stages to want to treat SARS as a local problem to be resolved locally. Partly, as stated above, this was due to the political and economic dynamics of Guangdong. Partly, it was due to the local perception that SARS could be brought under control. At that time, the number of people who had died from the outbreak was miniscule, almost negligible, compared to numerous others who have succumbed to more recurrent cases of influenza and respiratory problems often in the winter-spring period. Guangdong's Vice Mayor Chen Chuanyu was reported to have said in February 2003 that the disease was not as frightening as rumored. He added that the situation was under control and that it was completely possible to control and treat the disease.[16]

Likewise, the central authorities did not perceive SARS to be that serious a disease that warranted a national response. It was regarded as a

[14] While he was Party Secretary of Zhejiang, Zhang Dejiang was credited with creating a conducive environment for the private sector including small and medium-sized enterprises to flourish. As for Huang huahua, during his four year stint with the Guangzhou party committee, he earned a reputation as a reformist for helping oversee the remarkable transformation of Guangzhou into a modern metropolis.

[15] "Guangzhou new mayor vows to pursue growth goals", *South China Morning Post*, 30 Mar 2003.

[16] "The disease is not incurable, says vice-mayor. We can treat it. Guangzhou residents urged to ignore rumor-mongers", *South China Morning Post*, 12 Feb 2003.

medical issue best resolved by the relevant medical authorities. In early February 2003, a team of Beijing experts led by Deputy Health Minister Ma Xiaowei visited Guangdong to understand more about the disease.[17] In mid-February 2003, the Director of the Chinese Center for Disease Control and Prevention Li Liming was reported to have said that pneumonia was common and recurrent during the winter-spring period and could be attributed to many causes, and in this instance the causative agent was considered to be a curable disease. He further gave the assurance that there was no cause for panic.[18] In fact, one of the early findings by the Chinese Center for Disease Control and Infection, in collaboration with the Guangdong Center for Disease Control and Prevention, was that the cause of the outbreak was Chlamydia, a sexually-transmitted disease.[19] This was later found to be untrue.

It is difficult to ascertain how frequently and how much information the Guangdong authorities provided to authorities higher up on the SARS outbreak. The problem is unlikely to be one of accessibility since the Guangdong provincial government can report directly to the Political Bureau or other relevant central authority as Zhang Dejiang is a member of the Political Bureau. But it is clear that based on the information it was supplied with, the central authorities particularly the Ministry of Health either did not see the urgency or could not act quickly to contain the spread of the disease. To some extent, this could be attributed to the failure of the Guangdong authorities to fully inform the central authorities of the extent of the disease.[20] But more importantly, it showed the failure of the both the local and central authorities to appreciate how a local problem could snowball into a national issue.

[17] The visit took place on 9 Feb 2003.

[18] "Outbreak of pneumonia in Guangdong brought under control", *Xinhua News Agency*, 14 Feb 2003.

[19] "Cause of pneumonia outbreak in south China identified", *Xinhua News Agency*, 18 Feb 2003.

[20] According to Li Yiming, Director of Guangdong Health Information Coordination Center, at the height of the SARs crisis, it took eight to nine days to report a SARS case from the hospital located at the lowest administrative level to the Center for Disease Control in Beijing. See "Yue SARS shangbao xubatian" (To report a SARS case in Guangdong requires eight days), *Ming Bao*, 15 Nov 2003.

Another peculiar aspect of central-local relations worth mentioning here is that given the vast expanse of the country, the Beijing government authorities could not be fully relied on to curb the spread of SARS. While the central government can set guidelines and issue decrees, there is very little it can do to effectively help SARS-affected areas around the country. In several instances, local government officials initiated their own preventive measures to keep SARS away from their borders. In provinces such as Hebei, for instance, there was a serious shortage of different kinds of medical supplies. So to prevent SARS cases from being imported from Beijing, local officials took the drastic step of blocking the highway connecting Hebei and Beijing.[21] In other localities, local governments even temporarily suspended airlines flying in from Beijing. Even vehicles bearing Beijing licence plates were unwelcome in neighboring provinces and were told to turn back.[22]

Apart from the measures taken by the local government, residents of counties and villages would band together, either with or without the sanction of local government officials, to attempt to keep SARS at bay. Such actions can be attributed partly to inadequate understanding of the nature of SARS and partly to the lack of trust in the government's explanation of the extent of the outbreak. In mid-April 2003, when the Director of Health Bureau in Hangzhou (capital of Zhejiang) declared that there was no SARS cases in the city, public panic ensued. Many citizens were of the view that if the state says "no", it must be a "yes".[23] In provinces such as Zhejiang, Tianjin and Henan, rural residents demonstrated and protested to stop local governments from setting up quarantine centers for SARS patients.[24]

[21] Hebei, a province of about 65 million residents, has a large floating population who travel to Beijing regularly to find part-time work. See "Migrant workers aid outbreak in China", *Straits Times*, 8 May 2003.

[22] "Jingren zaobaiyan zheci zuidiulian" (Beijingers were frowned upon, this is the most embarrassing moment), *Ming Bao*, 19 May 2003.

[23] Personal phone conversations with Hangzhou residents.

[24] "Cunmin baoli kangshe geliying" (Villagers resort to violence to protest setting up of quarantine centers), *Ming Bao*, 6 May 2003. See also "Threat to China's social stability", *Straits Times*, 6 May 2003 and "Peasants riot against quarantine centers in 2 Chinese provinces", *Straits Times*, 6 May 2003.

To some extent, such acts of self-protection undertaken by rural residents is a reflection of the widening urban-rural divide, a hot topic among Chinese scholars. In the early stage of the reform and open-door policy, rapid economic development in the rural areas benefited the majority of Chinese peasants. But since the early 1990s, rural peasants have increasingly become an underprivileged social class. While the spurt in capitalistic development after Deng Xiaoping's southern tour in 1992 enriched lots of urban citizens, peasants found that the rural-urban divide has continuously enlarged. With more peasants migrating in search for a better life in urban cities, they found themselves being treated as second-class citizens by the urban citizens. Perhaps one of the serious shortcomings thrown up by the SARS episode is that rural peasants are virtually left out of China's healthcare system. With no healthcare support, the peasants could ill-afford to fall sick as they usually would not have enough money to see a doctor. As a result, peasants took matters into their own hands by setting up barricades at village entries to stop outsiders from entering their hometowns. They also protested against the setting up of quarantine centers in the vicinity of their households even though such centers were in their interests.

Third, bureaucratic fragmentation could also explain the government's poor and slow response to the SARS outbreak. Bureaucratic fragmentation is a universal phenomenon with each bureaucracy guarding its turf jealously and pursuing its own interests at the expense of others. To some extent, self-interested bureaucratic behavior played a role in the failure to contain the spread of SARS. In this case, fragmentation existed between the party's Department of Propaganda (DOP) and the MOH. Not only does the two belong to different organizational set-ups but there is also an inherent conflict of interest between the two.

The DOP, being the party's mouthpiece, has a predominant say over how information pertaining to SARS is managed.[25] Understandably, the

[25] As is well known, the DOP is one of the most conservative departments within the Party. In the 1980s, it initiated waves of political campaigns against so-called bourgeoisie liberalization. While the governmental structure has kept pace with the economic transformation of the country since the 1990s, the Party's various departments have remained intact.

interest of DOP is not to report on news which could impact negatively on the party's image. This was a consistent position adopted by the Guangdong provincial DOP and central DOP in Beijing. On the other hand, the MOH and Guangdong Bureau of Health as organs under the State Council, has to work within the parameters set by the party in general and specifically by the DOP in particular when dealing with information on the SARS outbreak. Logically, the MOH and Guangdong Bureau of Health would want to release as much information as possible on SARS and how it is transmitted so that preventive measures could be quickly put in place to contain the spread of the disease. Even assuming that this was what they wanted to see happen, they could not and did not attempt to move beyond the parameters set by the DOP. In other words, when it came to issues that mattered most, all government organizations are expected to fall in line with the position set by the party. In this regard, the DOP should share responsibility for the spread of SARS.

Fourth, the bifurcation of authority between the civilian government and the PLA impeded efforts to contain the spread of SARS. This division is equally, if not more serious, than the need for all government agencies to toe the line set by the DOP on information pertaining to SARS. In China, the military is virtually an independent kingdom onto itself, and the civilian government has difficulty in bringing the military under its control. Although in principle, the party commands the gun, in reality, even the party as an organization can hardly control the gun. Instead, it is individual leaders who can exert control over the military.

In Beijing, although there were a number of SARS cases in the military hospitals, these cases were meant to be kept secret and was not under the purview of the Beijing government or even the MOH. The military hospitals were not obliged to inform the civilian government of any information pertaining to SARS patients under their jurisdiction. Such a dichotomy between the military and civilian authority seriously impeded efforts to contain the spread of the disease. Each side went about its own way to attempt to contain the disease when the right approach would have been to pool resources and mount a joint effort. There was a brief but most embarrassing period when Beijing government officials downplayed the extent of the SARS outbreak. In the first press conference on SARS by a top official since the outbreak, Health Minister Zhang

Wenkang announced on April 3, 2003 that Beijing had reported 12 SARS cases and three deaths by the end of March.[26] He further provided the assurance that China was a safe place to "work, tour and live".[27]

It was clear to those well-informed that the figures provided by Zhang Wenkang on SARS cases in Beijing were grossly under-reported. They could not be so low if SARS cases in the military hospitals were included as purported by the Health Minister. One of them was Jiang Yanyong, a retired military doctor, who had followed developments closely and more importantly, was prepared to take action to correct the under-reporting. After his letter to CCTV and Phoenix TV to ask them to be forthcoming on the extent of the SARS outbreak in China was ignored, Jiang decided to go public himself with what he knew.[28] Jiang's disclosures triggered off greater international pressure and eventually forced the top leadership to take much more active interest on the SARS outbreak. From then onwards, there was much better coordination between the government and the military sectors.

All the aforesaid factors hastened the spread of SARS within and without China. In order to overcome the obstacles preventing a concerted national response and to restore China's credibility in the eyes of the world, Beijing's top leaders had to get involved. But taking action involved political risks. Although Hu Jintao was Party Secretary (since November 2002) and State President (since March 2003), he had yet to consolidate power. He had to tread carefully as Jiang Zemin was still Chairman of the Central Military Commission and as the majority of the Politburo Standing Committee members were either Jiang's men or Jiang's loyal supporters. It can be reasonably assumed that Hu had held consultations with Jiang on how the SARS outbreak could be best handled. But by the time SARS gripped the attention of the top

[26] "Ministry of Health releases data on distribution of SARS cases", *Xinhua News Agency*, 3 Apr 2003.

[27] "Health Minister — It is safe to live in China", *Xinhua News Agency*, 3 Apr 2003.

[28] Jiang Yanyong had first emailed his letter to CCTV and Phoenix TV (a pro-China TV station in Hong Kong) on 4 Apr 2003. After his e-mailed was ignored, Jiang was interviewed by Susan Jakes on 8 Apr 2003, a correspondent with *Time* magazine, which published the interview on the same day. See "Feature: A Chinese doctor's extraordinary April in 2003", at http://english.peopledaily.com.cn/200306/13/print20030613_118182.html.

leadership, mistakes had been made and there was little time to deliberate on the issue.

Hu Jintao therefore was in an unenviable position. On the one hand, being the ranking leader in China, he was expected to act quickly and decisively to diffuse the international furore and mounting domestic disquiet over China's lacklustre response to the SARS outbreak. This would include putting an end to the bouts of misinformation emanating from the relevant government authorities and punishing those who could be held accountable for the mistakes committed. Without an effective response, Hu's leadership at the helm of the party would be seriously questioned. On the other hand, Hu could not act without taking into account the prevailing political constraints. Failure to do so would mean alienating those whose support he is trying to win over to consolidate power.

On hindsight, there appeared to be some form of compromise reached between Hu Jintao and Jiang Zemin on how to contain the fallout from the SARS outbreak. It is perhaps worthwhile to recap that both Health Minister Zhang Wenkang and Beijing Mayor Meng Xuenong were removed at the same time.[29] Zhang was known to be a Jiang supporter, while Meng was perceived as Hu's protege. While the sacking of Meng was understandable because he had blatantly misled the public about the threat of SARS and failed to institute effective measures to prevent its spread, Meng's removal caught some observers by surprise.[30] They have concluded that Meng was made a sacrificial lamb by Hu to make it politically palatable for Jiang and his supporters to accept the demise of one of their members.[31] While this may be true, it is also possible that by removing two senior government officials, Hu was trying to limit the political damage to the party and not make too many enemies for himself. The real chief of Beijing, Liu Qi, Party Secretary and a member of the Politburo, got off with a public apology and remains in power. The downfall of Liu,

[29] They were both removed on 20 Apr 2003.

[30] Meng Xuenong was elected Beijing Mayor in January 2003 while Zhang Wenkang was appointed Health Minister in 1998.

[31] "Hu's political future may hinge on SARS", *International Herald Tribune*, 25 Apr 2003. See also "SARS battle puts new Chinese leader to the test", *The New York Times*, 26 Apr 2003 and "Pair sacked over handling of outbreak", *South China Morning Post*, 21 Apr 2003.

also linked to Jiang, would have dealt too hard a blow to Jiang's faction.

A week after the sacking of Zhang Wenkang and Meng Xuenong, Hu chaired a regular Politburo meeting to discuss the launching of a new round of study and implementation of the "Three Represents" theory.[32] The theory, enshrined in the party's constitution, is the essence of Jiang Zemin's legacy. A number of observers have wondered why Hu held a seemingly unrelated meeting during the critical period of combating SARS. How could the "Three Represents" theory provide an effective guide to the party leadership to combat SARS? It is hard to see any strong correlation between the two. But seen from the political perspective, Hu's gesture is of some significance. Hu was making use of the "Three Represents" theory to reach out to Jiang's faction and allay any concern that a political witch-hunt was in the offing. He wanted to show that he was for continuity and would work with Jiang's faction to combat SARS.[33]

At around the same time of the Politburo meeting, there appeared to be a closing of party ranks to deal with the SARS outbreak. Major figures in Jiang's faction including Wu Bangguo (NPC Chairman),[34] Huang Ju (Vice Premier)[35] and Jia Qinglin (Chairman of Chinese People's Political Consultative Conference)[36] came out to publicly exhort various sections

[32] "CPC to launch new round of study of 'Three Represents' theory", *Xinhua News Agency*, 28 Apr 2003.

[33] It is no coincidence that the same Politburo meeting discussed how to handle the relationship between economic work and the fight against SARS. The meeting also called on all localities and departments to continuously move forward with economic work while going all out to combat SARS.

[34] At the second meeting of the 10th NPC Standing Committee on 26 Apr 2003, Wu Bangguo called on all lawmakers to work closely with the central government to fight, SARS with the joint effort of all sectors. See "Chronology of China's fight against SARS since April 20 (7)", *Xinhua News Agency*, 30 Apr 2003.

[35] During an industrial tour in Beijing on May 2, 2003, Huang Ju stressed the importance of producing adequate SARS-related medical supplies and uninterrupted power supply to SARS-related hospitals and quarantined areas. See "Vice-Premier urges greater efforts to provide supplies for SARS fight", *Xinhua News Agency*, 2 May 2003.

[36] At a SARS workshop in Beijing on April 30, 2003, Jia Qinglin called for full multiparty cooperation by urging non-communist parties and individuals to devote themselves to the anti-SARS campaign. See "Non-communist parties asked to help fight SARS", *Xinhua News Agency*, 30 Apr 2003.

of the party, government and society to work together to fight SARS. Jiang himself issued an order to transfer a total of 1,200 military doctors and nurses from all major military units to Beijing hospitals designated to receive and treat SARS patients.[37] Although it was stated explicitly, it was clear that the party was rallying under the leadership led by Hu Jintao. Hu seemed to have scored a minor political victory.

STRENGTHS OF CHINA'S POLITICAL SYSTEM

The SARS outbreak has the tendency to show up weaknesses in the Chinese political system and underestimating its strong points. There are positive aspects of the Chinese political system in combating the SARS outbreak that are worth highlighting here. The most notable of which is that once SARS became a political issue and became an item on the national agenda, the top leadership accorded the highest priority to combat SARS. National resources were mobilized to deal with the outbreak. To a large extent, the authoritarian nature of the Chinese political system enabled the top leadership to implement quite effective measures to bring SARS under control.[38]

Once the top leadership decided that an all-out national effort was necessary, it moved quickly. The party made the first move and the government followed soon after. The Politburo Meeting chaired by Hu Jintao on April 17, 2003 on SARS was the first public indication that the top leadership was getting its act together. Three days later, Zhang Wenkang and Meng Xuenong were sacked. On April 23, 2003, Wen Jiabao announced the setting up of a national task force to combat SARS at a meeting of the Standing Committee of the National People's Congress. Vice Premier Wu Yi, an able assistant to former premier Zhu Rongji, was appointed commander-in-chief of the task force and subsequently made

[37] "Military medical staff transferred in emergency to Beijing for fighting SARS", *Xinhua News Agency*, 28 Apr 2003.

[38] The authors are not endorsing the authoritarian nature of the Chinese political system but are merely stating a fact.

Health Minister.[39] With an "iron lady" image and being highly regarded overseas, Wu Yi was deliberately selected to send a clear message to the domestic and international audience that China was serious about containing SARS.

Interestingly, a number of other new appointments with links to former premier Zhu Rongji were made. After Zhang Wenkang was removed, Gao Qiang, who worked for Zhu when the latter was premier from 1998 to 2003, was appointed Party Secretary of MOH. Wang Qishan, Governor of Hainan province, was summoned to Beijing and appointed Acting Mayor of Beijing, replacing Meng Xuenong. Wang, son-in-law of the late Yao Yilin (Politburo Standing Committee member and Deputy Premier), was also affiliated to Zhu Rongji. With these appointments, it would appear that the party and government under the Hu–Wen leadership was asserting its authority with the appointment of more professionally-minded officials.

But these personnel changes did not necessarily mean that Jiang and his faction did not support the Hu–Wen leadership. While Jiang's faction remains strong, it is not dominant in every aspect of Chinese politics. Most of Jiang's men are good at managing party affairs, not government affairs. On the other hand, most good technocrats are now located in the government sector, i.e., the State Council (SC) and its various bureaucracies. Under Zhu Rongji, the SC became a relatively less political cabinet, almost exclusively focusing on managing China's economy and other administrative matters. Most officials in the SC are professionals and technocrats. Hence, it should not be surprising that more of such technocrats would be pushed to the front in combating SARS. As mentioned above, Jiang and almost all the key figures from his faction showed their support to the Hu–Wen leadership in combating SARS.

It should also not be surprising that given the fragmented nature of China's political system and the distance between the centre and local levels of authority, the task of Beijing to ensure that local authorities do their job to combat SARS is not easy. Hence, what the top leadership did

[39] "China creates SARS task force, special fund", *Xinhua News Agency*, 23 Apr 2003. The deputy commander-in-chief of the task force was State Councillor and Secretary General of the State Council Hua Jiamin.

was to hold those in positions of authority accountable for their actions. With the removal of Zhang Wenkang and Meng Xuenong, a system of political responsibility was implicitly established. It had the effect of 杀鸡儆猴 (killing the chicken to frighten the monkeys). The underlining message was that henceforth any senior party or government official who is deemed to have failed in his duty to contain SARS under his area of jurisdiction could be removed. Indeed, within a short span of time, hundreds of government officials at different levels of government were removed for their dereliction of duty.

In Beijing city, after Wang Qishan's appointment, the leadership initiated various measures to deal with SARS, although many of them were regarded by outsiders as excessive. For instance, a special hospital for SARS patients, the Xiaotangshan Hospital, was built in less than ten days in a Beijing suburban area and was staffed with over 1,000 military doctors mobilized by the CMC. The hospital was a key part of Beijing's strategy to combat SARS by isolating SARS cases from the city to the suburban area.[40] The hospital was able to accommodate about 3,000 infected persons and this greatly lessened the burden on other hospitals. The mobilization of military doctors provided some relief arising from the shortage of doctors for contagious diseases control. For Beijing residents, they felt reassured that the city was a safe place to live in. Confidence in Beijing's municipal government also slowly returned.[41]

Apart from the urban areas, the top leadership was also concerned with containing the spread of SARS in the rural areas.[42] With no coverage under the healthcare system, rural peasants were more vulnerable to SARS than urban residents. It would be a political disaster if SARS

[40] After the SARS outbreak, the Beijing authorities found that the city was short of hospitals for infectious diseases and doctors. Several hospitals had to be used for SARS even though they did not have proper facilities.

[41] The Beijing authorities also set a goal for its officials that SARS had to be brought under control by the end of May 2003, a goal that was only achieved much later.

[42] After the collapse of the commune system in the late 1980s, rural healthcare system was virtually dismantled. The commune system under Mao Zedong had provided rural peasants some basic medical care and this played an important role in controlling different kinds of infectious diseases. Under that system, barefoot doctors were able to ply their trade to virtually every corner of the country.

where to spread out of control in the rural areas where the majority of the population lived. There had been reports that SARS-infected patients ran away from hospitals to avoid making medical payments. To deal with the issue, the top leadership declared that rural peasants, if infected, would receive free treatment and all costs would be borne by the state. This was a significant breakthrough as earlier calls by various cadres and social groups to accord peasants better treatment went on deaf ears. It showed that the Hu–Wen leadership was paying greater heed to the less privileged class as they had professed early in their term. The leadership also made great efforts to distribute medical equipments and necessary medicine to rural areas to help local governments combat SARS. In the event, SARS did not spread to rural areas, partly because of government policy and partly because of luck.

To contain SARS effectively, there was a need for the government to devise an effective legal framework to deal with the outbreak of public health emergencies. In line with this approach, the infectious disease act was amended to include SARS as an infectious disease.[43] More importantly, the amended law allows the death penalty to be meted out to those who intentionally spread the virus. In line with the infectious disease act, the State Council announced new guidelines in May 2003 to deal with emergency public health situations. The new guidelines clearly define the duty of relevant administrations in the event of the outbreak of a public health emergency and how such news should be reported. It also states that news of any public health emergency should be reported within 1–2 hours.[44]

It is worth noting that although SARS became an important item on the agenda of the Chinese leadership, it was not the only one. The

[43] When SARS was first discovered in Guangdong, it was treated as a local medical issue. Some government officials at that time attributed the delayed response to the fact that SARS was not listed then as an infectious disease. Since it was not an infectious disease, it should be dealt with by local government, not the central government.

[44] "Tufa gonggong weisheng shijian baogao youshixian: yidaoer xiaoshi" (The time limit to report on public health emergencies is 1–2 hours), at http://news.xinhuanet.com/newscenter/2003-05/12/content_866737.htm and "China improving legal system to cope with public health emergencies", *Xinhua News Agency*, 13 May 2003.

recognized the importance of paying equal attention to promote continuous economic development vital for political and social stability. Without sustaining a high growth rate, other problems such as unemployment, poverty and rural stability could worsen and threaten the stability of the country. In order to reduce the negative impact of SARS on China's economy, the leadership devised a two-pronged strategy of ensuring continuous economic growth while dealing with SARS (一手抓防治非典，一手抓发展经济).[45] From the perspective of the top leadership, SARS must not be allowed to slow down China's development momentum, otherwise there would be more problems.

Responding to External Pressure

The strength of China's political system could also be seen from its ability to make a complete change mid-way to deal head-on with the criticism levelled both internationally and domestically on China's lack of information provided and slow response to the SARS outbreak. Much of this change could be attributed to the changed perception towards the SARS outbreak held by the top leadership. Given China's weak institutional and legal framework, the role of the top leaders and their perception of the problems confronting the country would assume even greater importance. Once it was decided that it was no longer in China's interest to ignore the views of the international community and its own public, they began to react to contain the damage.

Initially, the regime adopted a non-cooperative attitude towards the World Health Organization (WHO) eager to conduct field trips to China to better understand the extent of the SARS outbreak.[46] It was also not receptive to comments from other countries calling on China to be more forthright on its SARS figures. Such criticisms were regarded as moves by the

[45] "Wen Jiabao zongli: gonggu chengguo fangfeidian fanfu, wuxiang cuoshi cuji jingji fazhan" (Premier Wen Jiabao: Consolidate measures to prevent the recurrence of SARS, five measures to spur economic growth), *Xinhuanet*, 5 Jun 2003.

[46] China's response was in stark contrast to that of the Vietnamese government which cooperated immediately and fully with the World Health Organization Office in Hanoi when SARS was first discovered in Vietnam.

foreign community to politicize the SARS outbreak, an ill-intentioned anti-China move. Nevertheless, with mounting international pressure and the rapid spread of SARS, Beijing leaders could no longer hold out from cooperating fully without serious damage to the image of the country and leadership.

Henceforth, there was a noticeable change in the government's attitude towards the international community. The government began to take steps to release more information on SARS and work with the international community to contain SARS. In late March 2003, the Chinese authorities issued updated data on SARS cases and deaths for the previously under-reported figures in Guangdong province, raising the cumulative totals from 305 to 792 and from 5 to 31 deaths. Also, under the leadership of Madam Wu Yi as Vice Premier and Health Minister, there was much closer cooperation between the Chinese government and WHO officials in terms of the daily reporting of SARS figures and accessibility to SARS affected areas in China.

At the international level, key Chinese leaders and officials went on a public relations drive to salvage China's tarnished reputation. When Wen Jiabao was invited to a specially convened ASEAN Summit on SARS in Bangkok in April 2003, he told his ASEAN counterparts that he had come in the spirit of "candid responsibility, trust and cooperation" and called for closer regional cooperation to fight SARS.[47] The Chinese government even went a step further to admit that mistakes were made in handling the SARS outbreak. At the World Health Assembly in Geneva in May 2003, Wu Yi admitted shortcomings in China's control of SARS and management of information related to the disease. She added that the inefficiency in some localities and departments have caused China's effort in controlling SARS to be "somewhat passive" for a period of time.[48] While on a Euro-Asian tour in May–June 2003, Hu Jintao

[47] See "Speech by Premier Wen Jiabao of China at the Special-ASEAN Leaders' Meeting on SARS, April 29, 2003", at http://www.fmprc.cn/eng/47989.html.

[48] See "Statement by Madame Wu Yi Head of the Chinese Delegation, Vice Premier and Minister of Health of the People's Republic of China at the General Debate of the 56th World Health Assembly, May 20, 2003", at http://www.fmprc.gov.cn/eng/49545.html. See also "Wu Yi: zhongguo yuan chengdan zeren, luxing yiwu yingdui yiqing" (Wu Yi: China is willing to take responsibility, carry out its duty to deal with SARS), *Xinhuanet*, 21 May 2003.

made the point in his meetings with other world leaders that the China was ready to cooperate extensively with the international community in the fields of public health and epidemic prevention.[49]

The much greater transparency displayed by the Chinese government was a breath of fresh air after months of avoiding addressing the subject head-on. The international community reacted by making positive comments about China's efforts in combating SARS.[50]

It is worth mentioning here a separate but related incident. At around the same time that China was more pro-active in combating SARS, *Xinhua News Agency* announced on May 2, 2003 that a Chinese Ming-class submarine that encountered a mechanical failure while on a regular training exercise left its crew of 70 officers and soldiers on board dead.[51] Included in the announcement was a condolence message to the victims' families and relatives signed by Jiang Zemin in his capacity as Chairman of the Central Military Commission.

Such an announcement was extremely rare in China as it had never been known to release news immediately after an incident occurred. And given that the submarine mishap was a purely military matter, not belonging to the public realm, the release of such news was significant. It would seem that the military, like the government, has become more sensitized to the need to be more transparent on issues which could have a serious political implication. It might not be too far-fetched to say that if the SARS episode had not forced the leadership to display more

[49] "Chinese president's Euro-Asian tour fruitful — FM", *Xinhua News Agency*, 5 Jun 2003.

[50] At their bilateral meeting in Evian in France in June 2003, President Bush praised Hu for his handling of the SARS crisis, especially his efforts to improve transparency. See "Bush invites Hu to pay a visit to Washington", *South China Morning Post*, 3 Jun 2003 and "Hu, Bush pledge to further develop constructive relations of cooperation", *Xinhua News Agency*, 2 Jun 2003.

[51] "Jiang Zemin fa yandian aidao 361hao qianting yunan guanbin weiwen qinshu" (Jiang issues condolence message to the relatives of officers and soldiers of the 361 submarine mishap), *Xinhua News Agency*, 2 May 2003, at http://www.chinanews.com.cn/n/2003-05-02/26/299688.html. See also "Seventy crew killed in submarine accident", *China Daily*, 3 May 2003 and "Suffocation killed 70 on sub, says report", *South China Morning Post*, 5 May 2003.

transparency, the PLA might not be so forthcoming with news of the Ming-class mishap. Regardless of the real motivation behind the decision to go public, a number of observers have already speculated that this could be an inkling of greater transparency to come on the part of the government and even party. But whether events would move in such a linear direction is a debatable point.

SARS and the Future of China's Political System

How will SARS affect China's political system? We have discussed the immediate impact of SARS on China's politics from the top to the bottom. Many observers have argued that SARS will push the leadership to initiate greater political liberalisation and even democratisation. As we have discussed, the SARS outbreak has shown up weaknesses in Chinese political system and thus highlighted what could be done to reform the system. There has also been pressure from both domestic social groups and the international community for the leadership to initiate some reform to improve the level of governance in the country. In some sense, the SARS outbreak appears to have created an unprecedented opportunity for the Hu–Wen leadership to undertake reform initiatives.

But the existence of conditions for political reforms does not necessarily mean that the leadership is prepared to or will initiate such reforms. In politics, there may not necessarily be a logical progression between prevailing conditions and possible outcomes. There are a number of factors that must be present before such a progression is possible. Foremost among them is that the leadership must have a strong willingness to engage in reforms. Apart from such an inclination, the leadership must have the capability to devise and implement reform policies. To examine the possible impact of SARS on China's political system, there is a need to pay particular attention to the orientations and thinking of the top leadership.

It is necessary at the outset to define what is meant by political reform. In the Chinese context, this term is not equivalent to the Western notion of liberal democracy where multi-party elections or checks and balances in the exercise of political power are norms. What the term does imply is that the Chinese top leadership reserves the right to experiment with various political reform initiatives that would strengthen the party's leading position in the country.

To be sure, talks about political reforms have gained momentum in the post-Mao period. Hu Yaobang, Zhao Ziyang and Jiang Zemin have initiated some degree of political reforms when they were at the helm. But attempts by both Hu Yaobang and Zhao Ziyang failed due to lack of strong political support for their reform initiatives. As for Jiang Zemin, he only embarked on his reform agenda in the latter half of his term with his "Three Represents" theory in February 2000. In his earlier years, Jiang's preoccupation was on consolidating power. Without a firm position, he could hardly engage in political reforms. Another reason why Jiang could avoid addressing political reform was that the tightening of the political atmosphere in the aftermath of the 1989 Tiananmen incident virtually frowned upon any form of political innovation.

Even though the political atmosphere has loosened somewhat today, Hu Jintao, in some sense, is facing a similar situation when Jiang was elevated to the top post years ago. Hu, like Jiang before, has to tread carefully to consolidate power. But unlike the Jiang Zemin era, the present leadership is likely to come under increasing pressure to initiate political reforms to accommodate the aspirations of a more diverse and complicated society.

Some observers have argued that Hu can consolidate his power by initiating political reforms using the opportunities created by the SARS outbreak. For instance, there was much hype in the media before July 1st that Hu is likely to introduce some reform measures during the anniversary celebrations of the founding of the party.[52] Also, in the immediate aftermath of the event, some media reports expressed disappointment that the expected political reforms did not materialize. *The New York Times*[53] and

[52] "Chinese leader solidifies power; defying predictions, President Hu raises hopes for significant political change", *The Washington Post*, 28 Jun 2003; "Hu speech likely to point way ahead", *South China Morning Post*, 30 Jun 2003; and "Hu speech likely to call for limited party reforms", *Straits Times*, 11 Jun 2003.

[53] "Analyst see tension in China within the top leadership," *The New York Times*, 1 Jul 2003.

International Herald Tribune[54] even suggested that Hu was unable to push ahead with political reforms because he was held back by Jiang and his supporters who fear that political change would usher in instability.[55]

While there could have been some tension between Hu and the supporters of Jiang over the issue of political reforms, it is most likely that Hu refrained from rocking the boat as he was still in an early stage of power consolidation. Any political reform is a risky enterprise since it involves the redistribution of power among different factions. Moreover, without securing strong support from Jiang Zemin and his faction, Hu is unlikely to initiate any political initiatives that would open him to criticism and undermine his authority.

While the existing power configuration rules out the possibility of any radical political reforms, some limited reforms are still likely, i.e., reforms with consensus that would not have any major negative impact on the distribution of power among factions. There appears to be a consensus among top leaders that China must be open to incremental political reforms in order to stay relevant to the needs of society.

In the short-term, the leadership is likely to focus its attention on the following areas. First is limited social and political transparency. As explained earlier, China's political system is generally regarded as one that lacks transparency. Before the SARS outbreak, the current leadership had already set a goal of improving the transparency of the political system. After Hu was elevated to the top post, he began to talk about limited media openness, i.e., allowing the media to report more on the

[54] "Hu signals a less reformist future in major speech, Chinese leader emphasizes Jiang's ideologies", *International Herald Tribune*, 2 Jul 2003. See also "Hu sticks to Jiang's theory in speech", *South China Morning Post*, 2 Jul 2003.

[55] James Mulvenon, who writes frequently for *China Leadership Monitor*, has suggested that Hu's July 1st speech reaffirms that despite the potential political opening offered by the governance crisis over SARS, Hu is unwilling or unable to directly challenge Jiang's leadership at this point in time, thereby portending more months of jockeying and ambiguity in the political arena and an unclear chain of command in the military realm. See James Mulvenon, "The crucible of tragedy: SARS, the Ming 361 accident, and Chinese party-army relations", *China Leadership Monitor*, No. 8, Fall 2003, http://www.chinaleadershipmonitor.org/20034/jm.html.

people and issues that affect their lives rather than primarily on the movements of the top leadership.

Within the Politburo, there have also been moves to make its proceedings more transparent. The meetings of the Politburo Standing Committee has been regularized and its agenda made known before each meeting. Also, party and government bodies are expected to make regular public announcements of decisions taken at closed-door meetings. Most significantly, during the third plenum of the 16th Party Congress in October 2003, Hu took the unprecedented step of submitting the Politburo's work report to the Central Committee and inviting them to give their comments. The party is willingly subjecting itself to limited political supervision. Hu appears to be placing emphasis on intra-party democracy. In other words, the pace of political reforms will continue to be set by the top. By extension, China is unlikely to bow or be seen to bow to external pressure to liberalize its political system.

The second likely outcome in the direction of political reform is to establish a limited system of political responsibility. Some efforts in this direction were already made in dealing with SARS. The removal of Zhang Wenkang, Meng Xuenong and other lower levels of government officials are signs that the leadership is keen to institute such a system. In June 2003, the CMC also fired Navy Commander Shi Yunsheng and Political Commissar Yang Huaiqing apparently for their responsibility in the Ming-class submarine mishap.[56]

However, given the fact that China will continue to be a one party system, such a political accountability system cannot be easily established. The removal of those who were negligent during the SARS outbreak could serve as a precedent to deal with errant officers who fail in their duties in the future, but this does not necessarily mean that the practice of political accountability will be established across the board. It would have to depend on the prevailing political circumstances and the judgement of the top

[56] "Jing zhongyangzhonggong pizhun, zhongyangjunwei fabu mingling tiaozheng haijun junzheng zhuguan" (Upon approval by Central Committee, the Central Military Commission issues order to reshuffle key military and political leaders in the Navy), *Xinhuanet*, 13 Jun 2003.

leadership of the risks involved. Moreover, a system of political responsibility requires a sound legal system which China lacks. It would take many years for such a system to be established and to function.

The third likely outcome in the direction of political reform is the willingness of the leadership to allow civil society to play a more important role to provide inputs in the decision-making process. The SARS outbreak has demonstrated that without cooperation from the civil society, the government will have great difficulty in managing a crisis. Under central direction, grass-roots communities played an important role in containing SARS, especially in places like Shanghai. Even rural peasants banded together on their own to combat SARS. While at times, these grass-roots groups might not necessarily see eye-to-eye with government policies, the government does realize the role that such social organizations played in containing SARS. On its own, the government would not have the means to cater to the specific needs of small communities or even individuals. Hence, there is value in adopting a decentralised approach to cope with emergencies at the people level.

In the medium term, the priority of the top leadership could be accorded to the following areas. The first is bureaucratic integration between different ministries and between central departments and local ones. Bureaucratic fragmentation at the top level delayed China's response to the SARS outbreak. The Chinese leadership since Deng Xiaoping has initiated waves of bureaucratic restructuring or rationalization. The SARS outbreak has highlighted the additional reforms that should be undertaken to deepen this reform agenda. The previous waves of reforms were aimed at accommodating a market economy with emphasis on restructuring economic bureaucracies. There might be a need to initiate more reforms and establish more mechanism to coordinate the work of different ministries or institutions. This is quite likely and is not an altogether a new practice. Already, the CCP's Central Committee has in place various so-called "small leading groups (SLGs)" (*lingdao xiaozu*) which comprised representatives from different backgrounds to better coordinate matters across ministries. But most of these SLGs have a specific focus and were established to cope with national "emergencies". Once a given emergency is over, the relevant group disbands. In some cases, the small leading groups even failed to perform its ascribed role. In this sense, the SLG system could be enhanced and more regular ones set up to monitor long term socio-economic trends and challenges.

Second, better coordination between the central ministries and the provinces also needs to be established. Although the central government continues to appoint major provincial leaders such as party secretaries and governors, Chinese provincial governments often operate like independent kingdoms. The linkage between the provinces and the central government is actually rather weak. Most of the time, the central government has to rely heavily on provincial leaders to provide necessary information since the country lacks an open and free media. In some cases, provincial governments may only provide the central government with selected information either based on their own political considerations or local interests. This may not be sufficient for the central government to arrive at an informed decision based on the information provided. Therefore, there might be a need to establish some effective mechanisms to coordinate provincial behavior.

A third area of possible improvement is in rural healthcare. The most difficult aspect of dealing with SARS was probably how to prevent SARS from spreading to rural areas. If SARS had spread to rural areas, then very little could be done to curb its spread. Rural areas do not have a good healthcare system. This was a factor behind the leadership's decision to provide free medical treatment for rural peasants if they were infected. Furthermore, having a good rural healthcare system is also of political significance. Poor peasants have less capacity to resist a natural disaster like SARS. When their survival is threatened, they are likely to take matters into their own hands and may even rebel. This is especially true in central China like Hebei, Hubei and Henan provinces where a tradition of rebellion is deeply rooted. It is no coincidence that during the SARS outbreak, Falun Gong again became very active in Hebei and this made the leadership sit up. An immediate crackdown was initiated. The SARS outbreak has highlighted once again how rural problems can easily develop into a social stability issue.

Rural problems such as poverty and peasants burden have troubled Chinese leaders for many years. Former premier Zhu Rongji tried to solve rural poverty problems but only scored partial success. The new leadership has also accorded high priority to rural issues. The leadership has decided to implement the "taxes for fees" (*fei gai shui*) system nationwide on an experimental basis, with the aim of reducing peasants' financial burden. And to establish a better rural healthcare system has also been an important agenda for the leadership for some years but no concrete measures have been implemented. The SARS outbreak has provided an opportunity for the new leadership to push ahead with reform in this area. The leadership has to take effective measures to implement the reform so that another crisis will not endanger social stability in rural areas.

The final question is whether in the long run there will be political democratization? The political road map ahead remains hazy and one would do well not to dwell too much on this point. We have discussed the short- and medium-term impact of SARS on China's political system. The above-mentioned limited political liberalization and reforms are likely since these are continuous efforts by the leadership to improve the existing political system and that these reforms are unlikely to have a major impact on the distribution of power among different factions.

On the other hand, democratization is a different matter altogether. Political liberalization might or might not lead to democratization. Democratization involves a redistribution of power; more importantly, it could bring about a new basis of legitimacy for the Chinese leadership. Its impact on China's political system will go beyond the political realm. At this juncture, it is too early and perhaps unrealistic to conclude that a crisis like SARS will lead to political democratization in China.

Chapter 3

Local Management of SARS in China: Guangdong and Beijing

LAI HONGYI

CENTRAL-LOCAL ARRANGEMENTS AND SARS MANAGEMENT

The SARS outbreak and local management in 2003 provide us a vivid case of observing central-local relations at work in China. The belated and weak response of Guangdong government toward the disease in the early months illustrates three profound problems in the relations. First, information asymmetry hampers prevention of SARS. Localities enjoy an advantage over information regarding local situation, and the state keeps sensitive information away from the public. The center often relies on the locals in the localities to supply information of the same kind. The state is also reluctant to publicize highly infectious diseases out of the fear of public panic, social instability, economic downturns, and political consequences. Second, the center has no comprehensive and sensible way of evaluating local officials' performance. It relies too much on quantitative or mechanical indicators. Until recent years it pays heavy attention to the growth rate of local economy, and recently it has paid some attention to major accidents and social protests as indicators of cadre incompetence. Third, local authorities need the central authorization before taking dramatic measures including mass mobilization, travel warning and quarantine to combat infectious diseases. As to be elaborated below, these central-local arrangements only invite officials to play down major natural catastrophes (including disease). This management had been encouraged by the center in the past. The result of the problematic central-local arrangement is weak and belated local responses to diseases.

At the second stage of the SARS management, China's national government acted decisively. It utilized its administrative control of local cadres, improved gathering of information from localities and disclosure of SARS information and situation, and actively coordinated bureaucracies and localities in SARS management. This largely constructive change in the interaction of the center and localities helped China to keep SARS under control within two months.

INSTITUTIONAL PROBLEMS IN EARLY SARS MANAGEMENT

Three problems characterized central-local relations in China. They were: (1) information asymmetries in favor of the lower-level bureaucrats and against higher-level leaders and in favor of the state and against the public; (2) mechanical and one-sided evaluation of cadres' performance; and (3) fragmented bureaucratic authority. These three problems led to ineffective SARS management in the early months.

Information Asymmetries

Accurate information is vital for operation of any organization. This is particularly true for a government. The Chinese regime of information has two conventional characteristics — information asymmetries first in favor of lower-level bureaucrats and secondarily in favor of the state. First, higher levels of the Party and government bureaucracy rely heavily on lower levels to report various types of information, including local disasters, diseases, and outstanding problems. This gives local officials and lower-level bureaucrats an edge in information *vis-à-vis* their superiors. Second, the Chinese state has been suppressing sensitive information. This gives the state, or officials, an edge in information concerning the political, economic and social state of the country and its external standings over the common people.

Information edge at the lower level. Both asymmetries have their drawbacks. A major drawback of local information asymmetry is that national leaders are deprived of alternative sources of information. They have to rely on information transmitted from the bottom up inside the political system or bureaucracy. At each layer, bureaucrats who transmit the information have an incentive to distort it in order to protect their own careers. As a Chinese popular saying suggests, a typical approach adopted by Chinese officials *vis-à-vis* their superiors is *bao xi bu bao you*, namely, to report the good news and suppress the bad news.

Chinese officials dare to distort the information out of two calculations. First, the center relies on them to report information and has difficulties in developing alternate sources. The center would have to commit plenty of manpower and resources in order to produce an alternate source simply for any ad hoc case. This will be very costly and cannot be done for a large number of cases. The result is that the center falls back on localities for first-hand information and that the center has difficulties in finding out whether local officials distort the facts. Second, even if the center knows local cadres lie, it still has to rely on them to implement its own orders. It will be relatively lenient in penalizing them

Chinese officials, who are used to the autocratic information control, can be quite hostile to and ready to suppress any alternate source of information. Huang (1996, 228) pointed out that many Chinese officials feared negative media publicity more than administrative and political censure, because negative publicity could put an end to their own careers once for all. Open media criticisms can inflict greater damage on an official's career than administrative censure, and they can err. In this sense, administrative censure can be gentler and humane. However, administrative censure can be effective only when reliable information is available for higher-level officials, and this is not easy in China given the above analysis. As a result, administrative censure is rarely used and is hardly effective in correcting mistakes in official conduct. The result, as Lieberthal (1995, 175) vividly put, is self-defeating for the Chinese state: "Beijing's determination not to allow people to criticize the government has led to a policy of suppressing all independent sources of information gathering and transmittal, such as a free press. By thus denying themselves the one relatively systematic option for checking the accuracy of the information they receive, the top Chinese leaders have made themselves virtual captives of their own system and of the distortions it inevitably produces."

State's information control. The Chinese state monopolizes vital information regarding the regime and pending crises. This can be highly useful for the state. It can suppress most or even all the negative news about its performance, its external environment, and the scale of disasters in a given region. By feeding the population mainly good news, it can instill a high-level of confidence in the populace.

However, this practice has two critical drawbacks. First, in many cases the public can take necessary action to prevent the disaster only when it is informed. Suppressing negative information can only aggravate the disaster. Informing the public may lead to certain public panic in the short turn, yet may induce it to behave in a rational fashion over a protracted period to avoid the disaster. Second, should the state suppress the information regarding a pending crisis and eventually fail to prevent it, the populace will be discontented over the state's performance. The state may lose credibility and even legitimacy.

To be sure, in the past two decades, the Chinese media has undergone considerable changes and has been much more commercialized than before. Since the early 1980s, with the gradual cut in subsidies and emphasis on self-financing, news media in China has become increasingly commercialized and grown in number. The number of newspapers grew from 186 in the mid 1980s at the beginning of reform to 1,800 around 2000, that of magazines from several hundreds to over 7,000, and that of TV stations from 700 to around 9,000. Private capital entered the market, media competition has also intensified, distribution monopolies have broken down, and the media has become more pluralistic. Since the 1990s, news on web has been also attracting a growing number of readers (Stevenson-Yang, 2003, 223–231). In addition, short messages on cell phones also transmit news and sometimes rumors.

Nevertheless, the state's information control remains. It has lessened its control over politically less sensitive subjects, such as international news, leisure, entertainment, sports, technology, shopping, marriage and family, and low-level official corruption. However, it has maintained its tight control over sensitive issues. Two ministries play a particularly important role in keeping a political bridle over the media. The first two are the Propaganda Department of the Chinese Communist Party (PDCCP) and the State Press and Publications Administration (PPA).

The PDCCP formulates regulations and policies over the media and issues directives on how the media should cover issues of core importance or ad hoc sensitive issues. It also hires groups of retired editors in the cities to read newspapers and magazines to see whether its contents have confirmed to stated policies or not. It can remove editors of newspapers, magazines and TV stations. The PPA has staff members reading popular national news outlets and can stop publication without notice. Publications are subject to pre- as well as post-publication review by national or local propaganda authority. In addition, propaganda authorities held monthly meetings on ideological contents with publications. On these "blowing-the-wind" meetings, officials tell the latter how to cover hot topics and what to avoid (Stevenson-Yang 2003, 232–239).

During the SARS outbreak, national leaders also relied heavily on local officials for information, especially regarding the nature and effects of the disease. Vital information on SARS in Guangdong took quite a long time to reach the center, and its accuracy was reportedly questionable. In mid December 2002, two SARS patients sought treatment in Heyuan City. They infected eight medical workers. Around the New Year Day the Guangdong authority learned about the infectious disease. In early January, public health experts in Guangdong studied the disease in Heyuan and concluded that this was a new lung disease. SARS broke out again in Zhongshan on January 2, 2003, infecting over 12 patients and nine medical workers. Leading epidemic experts in the province surveyed the outbreak in late January and concluded that this was an unusual pneumonia. The provincial public health bureau was aware of these outbreaks.[1] Only around the end of January, upon seeing the rapid spread of SARS, Guangdong leaders felt impossible to hide it from Beijing. They then wrote a report to the Politburo, reporting only 600 cases and placing the other half of the cases under the category of suspect cases. They also recommended that the center should black out news reports on the

[1] He Li. 2003. *SARS Tests China (SARS Kaoyan Zhongguo)*. Beijing: Renmin Chubanshe, p. 7; "An inside story of how Guangdong discovered atypical pneumonia: Lin Jinyan fired the first shoot of the campaign of fighting AP", posted at http://www.sina.com.cn on 28 Apr 2003, accessed on 3 Jun 2003.

disease in order to pre-empt the outside world from attacking China and stabilize the situation.[2]

In addition, initially local and later national authorities were slow in providing information. Local authority in Guangdong suppressed news about SARS. Following a small SARS outbreak in Heyuan and news blackout in late December 2002, exaggerated rumors about the mysterious disease and the death of three medical workers circulated in Heyuan in early January 2003. Many people lined up to buy antibiotics. In the fist week of January, Heyuan officials tried to calm the local populace by denying the existence of the disease on local newspaper and meetings. While social chaos was prevented, a valuable opportunity for transmitting the information to higher authority, for alerting the public, and for stemming the spread of the disease might have missed.[3] Thus, the disease surfaced again in Zhongshan and Guangzhou.

Guangdong has been a bridgehead in commercialization in China. Its media is among the most commercialized in the country. It has also the most the outspoken and widely-read newspapers in the country, *Southern Weekend (Nanfang Zhoumuo)* with over one million circulations, *Southern Urban Post (Nanfang Dushi Bao)*, and *Goat City Evening Posting (Yangcheng Wanbao)*. In early February, following the above suggestion by Guangdong authority to suppress information, the PDCCP issued a directive, stipulating that reports on SARS should follow official uniform formats, data, approach, and style and should emphasize that it was under control.[4] The propaganda department's ban on reports prevented local residents from obtaining relevant information from local newspapers.

Eventually, the public started also to realize about the rapid spread of the disease. Between February 8 and 10, countless messages were transmitted through cell phones, internet and telephones regarding the disease. The people believed it was deadly and rushed to buy *banlangeng* (a Chinese medicine against the cold), vinegar (believed to kill gems),

[2] "The truth of Guangdong suppressing epidemic situation and cracking down on the media", posted at www.boxun.com on 14 May 2003, accessed on 3 Jun 2003.

[3] "A complete story of Guangdong's encounter with atypical pneumonia", posted at http://news.beelink.com.cn on 12 Feb 2003 ,accessed on 3 Jun 2003.

[4] News report by Xia Wensi, posted at http://www.boxun.com on 14 May 2003.

antibiotics, masks, and salt. Prices of these items even soared by ten or dozens of times.

Referring to the PDCCP directive, the Guangdong authority tightened media reports on SARS and cracked down on media that had openly discussed the disease. Reportedly, the News Office of Guangdong Propaganda Department issued as many as three prohibitive notices a day when SARS was rampaging Guangdong. On February 11, Guangdong held the first press conference on SARS, disclosing 305 cases and five deaths and declaring it was brought under control. Starting from March, it cracked down on the outspoken newspapers in Guangdong. It replaced the editor of *Southern Weekend*.[5]

The suppression of vital information had helped Guangdong to retain economic prosperity in one of the busiest shopping and tourism seasons. However, it deprived the populace and especially patients, their relatives, and medical workers of an opportunity to take extra precaution against a highly infectious and deadly virus. The disease continued to spread within and outside Guangdong through patients, their social contacts and medical professionals. Despite an earlier outbreak in Heyuan, the disease continued to rampage Zhongshan and later the provincial capital Guangzhou.

Information on SARS in Beijing was provided by both the Health Ministry and Beijing Government. Beijing leaders first learned of SARS in the city in the early March. However, due to the coming sessions of the National People's Congress and the Chinese People's Political Consultative Conference, the news was suppressed. The Beijing authority wanted to ensure that the two sessions would be held at a peaceful, calm, and successful atmosphere. After the sessions were over, Beijing officials continued to hide local SARS conditions.

Until early April, the Health Ministry continued to insist that Beijing was safe and SARS had little effect on the city. On April 3, Health Minister Zhang Wenkang declared that there had been only 12 SARS patients and three deaths. The WHO, however, did not trust the statistics provided by the Health Minister and Beijing Government.

[5] "The truth of Guangdong suppressing epidemic situation and cracking down on the media", *ibid.*

It took Dr. Jiang Yanyong's and other insiders' testimony to forcefully expose the fallacies in the official statistics. On April 8, *Time* magazine published a letter by Dr. Jiang. He testified that No. 309 military hospital alone had admitted 60 SARS patients, and seven of them had died. When the WHO team inspected Beijing in mid April, a military hospital (No. 309 Hospital) moved over 40 SARS patients to a hotel, and China-Japan Friendship Hospital put 31 pneumonia patients on ambulances running around the city. They played these tricks to evade WHO's attention.

Cadre Performance Assessment

In the reform era, official performance has been judged primarily by their abilities to generate local economic development and maintain social stability. As growth rates are a readily available indicator of economic growth, they become the surrogates for local official performance indicators. The national authority apparently emphasized social stability in evaluating cadres out of the following probable reasons. First, panic, rush buying, and other socially disrupting acts can threaten social stability. It may escalate into political outbursts and protests that target at the state. In addition, it could hurt economic growth, worsen unemployment and poverty, and in turn, create social forces discontented over the state's performance.

The state emphasizes economic growth in evaluating local cadres' performance out of the following reasons. First, out of a great variety of indicators, economic growth is the easiest and most sensible one. Other indicators may bias toward one group of provinces. For example, the level of public health and life expectancy may bias toward developed provinces that had more hospitals and more qualified doctors.

Second, economic growth can help solve the most pressing social problems in China, including unemployment, income, poverty, and backwardness. Job creation, in particular, constitutes an acute problem for national leaders. The job situation in the cities was bleak. In the third quarter of 2002, for example, the ratio of laborers needed and job seekers reached 0.78; unemployed made up 59% of the job seekers; and people aged 16 to 34 constituted 70% of total job hunters in 89 cities. Registered urban unemployed in September 2002 totaled 7.5 million, a 0.44 million gain from the end of 2001. This placed the official urban unemployment rate at 3.9%, a 0.3% increase from the end of 2001. In several relatively developed counties, urban unemployment rate reached a double digit. In addition, a large population of rural laborers is seeking jobs in the cities (Mo 2003, 35–39). Should high unemployment, especially among the young continue, violent crimes may multiply. Under this context, rapid economic growth generated a large number of jobs, easing already serious unemployment problems (Mo 2003, 41).[6] Therefore, national development plans since the early 1990s always set a target of high annual growth rate above 7%.

Central preference for growth has encouraged local leaders to induce and maintain economic development within their tenure. Some scholars, such as Gore (1998), even characterize local leaders' behavior as bureaucratic entrepreneurialism. Two reasons accounted for this behavioral trait. First, as Huang (1996) amply demonstrated, the national authority retained its final say in appointing provincial-level leaders. Provincial leaders, in turn, appoint lower-level local leaders. Second, localities draw their economic plans based on national growth targets (Gore 1998, 106–108). The end result is that a high growth rate can impress local leaders' superiors and increase an official's chance for promotion. On the contrary, an obvious failure for local leaders to meet the target can be easily interpreted as incompetence and may lead to setbacks in their careers.

In a similar vein, the local as well as national government devoted scant resources to public health. Public health was viewed as an unproductive area for public spending, and would consume valuable funds that could have directly stimulated economic growth. Public health is thus seriously under-funded. Nor did local and national governments pay sufficient attention to public health. In a populous country like China, infectious diseases are numerous and frequent. Partly for this reason, the government is slow to act on and take high-profile and drastic measures on infectious diseases.

In recent years, the center mandates localities to report any accidents that involved over a few deaths. The State Council under Premier Zhu introduced this stipulation in order to curb a rising number of accidents

[6] Refer to Lieberthal (1995, 244–245) for more discussion of national leaders' incentives for high growth.

and a large number of deaths each year. While this stipulation might have helped to penalize potential responsible cadres, it may have one unintended consequence. Since any leading cadre will be responsible for any major accidents involving three or more deaths and since each year such accidents are numerous in the provinces, this stipulation may unnecessarily punish leading cadres for accidents that are beyond their control. Cadres may hide or under-report accidents in order to evade their genuine or falsely-assumed responsibilities.

SARS, even when it first surfaced, appeared to be a mysterious and highly infectious disease. Publicizing the disease would definitely cause local residents to stay home and avoid shopping, dining, and traveling. It would also prompt outsiders, including tourists and business people, to avoid traveling to the locality. In the short-term, it will cause a downturn in the local and even economy. Therefore, publicizing the disease would potentially reduce the chance for localities and the nation to achieve their high growth targets and aggravate already serious unemployment problems. That is why local leaders preferred to hide the news about the disease. Even when they gave notice about the disease, they intentionally kept it vague.

Upon learning the infectiousness of the disease, Guangdong public health officials issued a belated and vague warning to all hospitals and public health officials in the province. Although it mentioned the unknown and infectious pneumonia, it was vague about its highly infectious nature and short of clear, effective, and drastic measures to prevent the disease from spreading. The notice was issued around January 21. However, public health and provincial officials kept the warning off many concerned officials until the end of the Chinese New Year holiday around February 7. An official at Guangdong public health bureau explained two reasons for this decision. First, the Chinese New Year, the largest holiday and happiest time for the Chinese, was coming. A health warning would cause panic. Second, the Chinese New Year was also the biggest shopping season of the year. Should the warning be clear and alerting, the public would stay home and avoid travel, shopping, and dining, and the economy would suffer drastically. At a close door meeting, a vice governor of Guangdong criticized Hong Kong's open coverage of the disease for hurting the economy and causing social panic. She reportedly say: "You can see how much trouble the Hong Kong government created for itself after it made everything public. They didn't have the ability to control and handle the disease, so what good was it to make everything public? Their tourism and investment are affected. Most of all, their people are in chaos. What a great loss."[7]

As stated, the state requires local leaders to report accidents that involve three or more deaths. Guangdong's local and provincial leaders might have under-reported SARS in order to avoid blames for major accidents in their jurisdiction.

In Beijing, the local government and probably the Health Minister initially suppressed the news about SARS in order to assist the smooth going of NPC and PCC sessions. Later on these officials, along with hospital officials, under-reported statistics on SARS probably in order to convey to the center a good impression about their performance. The hospitals might also want to ensure patients will keep coming to them, and publishing the news would hurt their business and profits.

Fragmented Authority

China scholars have noticed that the decision making power in China tends to be divided by fragmented institutions. Earlier literature points to the cleavage of institutions between the center and locale, and parallel vertical bureaucratic systems and dual leadership.[8] Lieberthal even coined the Chinese political model "fragmented authoritarianism".[9] The Chinese government, both national and local, as well as its health agencies, suffered from poor coordination and communication. First, there is very poor communication within the public health system in a province as developed as Guangdong. In addition, communication between localities within a province (Guangdong in this case) is also seriously insufficient. When SARS broke out and infected eight medical workers in Heyuan in late December, most hospitals in Zhongshan and Guangzhou were in the dark and took no precaution against it. Some hospitals did

[7] "China's slow reaction to fast-moving illness," posted at http://www.washingtonpost.com on 2 Apr 2003, accessed on 4 Apr 2003.
[8] See Lieberthal and Oksenberg, 1988.
[9] See Lieberthal, 1992.

gain valuable first-hand information in treating the disease. But due to poor communications and institutional setup, they did not share the information with colleagues in other hospitals. For example, the Heyuan hospital soon introduced quarantine, prevented further spread of the virus, and cured the infected medical workers. In December, the First Hospital of Guangzhou Medical School treated the SARS patient from Heyuan and gained insights into the disease. Dr. Zhong Nanshan, who oversaw the treatment, reported the disease to the Disease Control Station of Yuexiu District of Guangzhou. From mid January onward, 13 medical workers in Zhongshan were infected by SARS patients. Around January 21, Guangdong public health authority came to realize this highly infectious disease, and issued a vague warning to local health authorities and hospitals in the province, warning them of the disease and informing them of preventive measures. Still, many medical workers did not realize the effective measures against infection, and fell prey to the disease one after another. Major hospitals in Guangzhou repeated the same tragedy in Heyuan and Zhongshan.[10]

Second, there is a lack of information sharing between military and civilian hospitals. In Guangdong, after January 31 several military hospitals in Guangzhou treated SARS patients. The Guangzhou Air Force Hospital had no infection by the patients. Apparently it had been well aware of the infectiousness of the disease and implemented effective treatments. However, civilian hospitals in Guangzhou did not share its valuable information. As a result, SARS patients infected scores of medical workers in several large hospitals in Guangzhou in February. Only after paying for costly tuition did these hospitals come to know on their own how to protect their staff and prevent infections within the hospitals.

Third, public health and military institutions across provinces did not exchange vital information.[11] Even though initially military hospitals and then civilian hospitals in Guangzhou understood how to prevent infections by SARS patients in February, military hospitals (such as Nos. 301 and 302 hospitals) in Beijing also repeated the costly learning

[10] "Blocking action", posted at http://news.xinhuanet.com on 22 Apr 2003, accessed on the same date.

[11] "Instructions in February may have been a culprit in the extensive spread of SARS", posted on http://www.chinesenewsnet.com on 6 Jun 2003, accessed on 7 Jun 2003.

curve from early March onwards and experienced rapid spread of SARS within the hospital. In addition, in the early months of SARS outbreak, provinces whose rural workers and business people traveled frequently to Guangdong learned nothing about the disease in Guangdong. They did not alert their residents about the danger of traveling to Guangdong. Nor did they prepare their health officials and medical workers for the disease. As a result, some of them were hit by the rapid and serious spread of the disease in the following weeks.

Fourth, Guangdong failed to notify Hong Kong in time about the seriousness of SARS. This secrecy was to a considerable extent responsible for the rampage of SARS in Hong Kong. The Guangdong health authorities first informed their Hong Kong counterparts about the SARS epidemic in mid-February.[12] However, as the official media in Guangdong and China's public health minister stressed that SARS was under control, the health authority and hospitals in Hong Kong let off their guard. They were also under the illusion that Guangdong, a developing economy with questionable personal sanitary habits and inadequate health facilities, was prone to the disease, but not Hong Kong. The Hong Kong health chief also ignored warnings about SARS from health experts.[13] When Hong Kong hospitals received the first stream of SARS patients who contracted it in Guangdong, medical professionals were ill prepared. Even when they were told about this deadly and contagious illness, few believed and took precaution. This led to a high rate of within-hospital infections and afterwards widespread infection within residential communities.[14] Guangdong established formal direct contact mechanism on health issues with Hong Kong only on April 11, after SARS had spread in Hong Kong and other parts of the world. [15]

[12] "HK alerted one month after Guangdong case", posted on http://straitstimes.asia1.com.sg on 13 Jun 2003, accessed on the same date.

[13] "Hong Kong erroneously believed Zhang Wenkang", posted at http://www.mingpaonews.com on 21 Apr 2003; "Yang ignored three warnings and missed best opportunities for quarantine", posted at http://www.mingpaonews.com on 23 Apr 2003.

[14] "China's slow reaction to fast-moving illness", posted at http://www.washingtonpost.com on 2 Apr 2003, accessed on 4 Apr 2003.

[15] "HK alerted one month after Guangdong case", posted on http://straitstimes.asia1.com.sg on 13 Jun 2003, accessed on the same date.

Finally, Guangdong alone did not have the full formal authority to mobilize various branches of provincial bureaucratic agencies, such as transportation, aviation and borders to fight SARS. Formally, these provincial bureaucratic agencies would obtain approval and clearance from their national offices. In late April, when these agencies were mobilized to fight SARS, directives of individual agencies were issued by their national offices.

However, Guangdong leaders still have informal power to direct these branches and coordinate their activities in the province. For example, Guangdong public health authority could investigate the disease and issued warnings to health departments and hospitals in the province. Therefore, this lack of formal provincial coordinating power did hamper, but would not have prevented Guangdong from fighting SARS if its leaders decided to do so.

In Beijing, the military and civilian systems appeared to have a problem in communication at the early stage. SARS statistics in the military hospitals probably bypassed civilian leaders and were reported to military health authority and probably Jiang Zemin, the Chairman of the Central Military Commission. Premier Wen was said to complain that the military hid relevant statistics from him.[16] Vice Health Minister Gao admitted that the early SARS counts did not include 235 patients in the military hospitals.[17]

Central-Local Relations at the Second Stage of SARS Management

From early April onward, national leaders, especially Hu Jintao and Wen Jiabao, realized the increasing danger of mishandling SARS. They acted to mobilize the political machinery (the Party and the administration including public health agencies), social organizations, and the people to fight the disease. The center played up three instruments, injected new (even if temporary) dynamics into central-local relations, and eventually help turn secretive and low-profile SARS handling into open and effective management.

[16] News report from http://www.chinesenewsnet.com.com on 13 May 2003.

[17] "China admits underreporting its SARS cases", posted at http://www.nytimes.com on 21 Apr 2003, accessed on the same day.

Centralized Control of Cadre Careers

As Huang (1996) suggested, the Chinese national authority retained its administrative control of cadres. At the second stage of SARS management, national leaders applied this reserved weapon to cope with the runaway epidemic. It ordered cadres to act forcibly on SARS, held them responsible for the outcome, and penalized ineffective senior officials. They also gave a green light for all localities and institutions to pick and punish disobedient and incompetent officials in SARS management.

On April 13, Premier Wen called on officials to take decisive and effective measures to contain SARS. On April 17, State President and Party Secretary Hu Jintao chaired a Politburo Standing Committee meeting. The meeting stressed that fighting SARS was an important task and that leaders at all levels should command the fight and should disclose truthfully the epidemic statistics.[18] On April 20, 2003, two ministerial-level officials, namely, Public Health Minister Zhang Wenkang and Beijing Mayor Meng Xuenong, were removed from their posts, apparently for their inabilities to keep SARS under control. The decision on April 17 and dismissals of these two senior officials on April 20 amounted to a call for urgent action as well as a stern warning to all bureaucratic, provincial, and local leaders. It signaled to them that: (1) either they followed the national order to fight SARS, or they would a free fall in and even end to their political careers; and that (2) they were held responsible for the conditions of SARS in the localities or work units under their jurisdiction. As a result, Party branches and bureaucracies singled out and swiftly penalized incompetent and disobedient cadres. Since mid April, thousands of cadres from provincial down to village-level officials were relieved of their posts or disciplined due to their inabilities to manage SARS.[19]

As a result of central pressure, national ministries and all localities quickly switched to high gear to manage SARS, disclosed more reliable

[18] "Hu Jintao chaired Politburo Standing Committee meeting — No cover-up of atypical pneumonia situation is allowed", posted at http://www.sina.com.cn on 17 Apr 2003, accessed on the same date.

[19] "How to form enduring mechanism to reward and punish cadres in unusual circumstances", posted at http://news.xinhuanet.com on 26 Jun 2003, accessed on 10 Oct 2003.

statistics, isolated patients and suspected patients, and tried hard to stem the spread of the disease. In return, the center became better informed about the epidemic situation in the localities and could better handle the crisis.

The dismissals of two officials affected Beijing more than Guangdong. Despite criticisms from Hong Kong and on the Internet, leaders in Guangdong were intact. In addition, the peak for SARS has passed in Guangdong. In Beijing, Party Secretary Liu Qi assumed the directorship of a small group for preventing and treating SARS. Wang Qishan became the acting mayor. He quickly accelerated efforts to fight SARS. More reliable SARS statistics were updated and published daily. On April 20, the number of SARS patients in Beijing jumped from originally reported 37 to 339, plus 402 suspected cases. Beijing stood out as the second epicenter of SARS in mainland China after Guangdong. To contain the rapidly spreading SARS, a large and special hospital (Xiaotangshan Hospital) for infectious disease was quickly built in the suburb. It housed 1,000 beds. Institutions and many residential communities where SARS patients were discovered were quickly closed and cordoned off. Many entertainment centers were closed. Beijing also prohibited universities and schools from organizing group tours during the Labor Day holidays.

National Co-ordination and Supervision

Shortly before and after the Politburo's decision to fight SARS, several national ministries issued directives to their branches, urging them to take measures to prevent the spread of the virus. On April 14, the Ministries of Health, Finance, Railway and Transportation and the Bureau of Civil Aviation jointly issued an announcement to stem the spread of SARS through public transportation. They asked their local branches and local governments to look out for passengers suspected of SARS at stations of public transportation, isolate and treat them timely, and sanitize these places. The following day, the State Administration for Quality Supervision and Inspection and Quarantine and the Ministry of Health jointly issued an announcement, stepping up the health inspection of people crossing the border and urging to immediately send suspected patients to hospitals. On the same day, the Ministry of Health ordered all local branches to report SARS statistics each day. Two days later, on April 17, the Ministry of Health, together with the State Administration for Tourism, issued a program, directing tourist agencies how to contain SARS.[20] These policies by national ministries and bureaus paid the way for local branches to take necessary action to control the disease. However, one may suspect that without the national order to fight SARS, how far and how sincerely local governments and local branches of these ministries would enforce these necessary measures. As stated above, provincial and local leaders answered to their superiors, not these ministries. Therefore, only the national Party and administration (the State Council) could pressure them to take the issue seriously and act sincerely on it.

After mid April, the central leaders finally took the lead in enforcing and coordinating SARS management among bureaucratic agencies, among provinces, and between provinces and Hong Kong. As stated, on April 17, the Politburo Standing Committee ordered localities to treat SARS as one of the most important tasks. Three days later, they dismissed two senior officials and warned all officials to take the issue seriously. On April 23, the State Council formed a command center for preventing and curing atypical pneumonia (ATP). Vice Premier Wu Yi, who took over as Health Minister on April 20, was appointed as the director. A fund for preventing and curing ATP, totaling 2 billion yuan, was established on April 23.[21] The national government ordered all provincial and ministerial leaders to stay in their posts to fight SARS and avoided overseas travels. It authorized provincial Party and administrative leaders to command the health agencies under their jurisdiction and mobilize all necessary resources.[22] It sent out inspectors throughout the country to supervise local efforts and implementation.

Under the central leadership and pressure, many localities formed a coordinating agency to handle SARS and local leaders personally took

[20] News reports posted at http://news.sina.com.cn between 14 and 17 Apr 2003.

[21] "Uniformly coordinating the nation's prevention and curing: China established a command center for fighting the infectious disease", posted at http://www.zaobao.com on 24 Apr 2003, accessed on the same day.

[22] "Provincial and municipal leaders stay to fight the infectious disease and not allowed to go overseas", posted at http://www.mingpaonews.com on 23 Apr 2003, accessed on the same date.

charge. Hospitals were mobilized and equipped as permitted by local resources, transportation hubs were inspected and sanitized, and suspect patients were detected and in many cases, received immediate treatment. In a couple of months, SARS was brought under control.

In Guangdong, between mid and late April, several local bureaus of national ministries took precautionary measures. Hospitals in Guangzhou established special rooms to treat patients with fever. Elementary and high schools were asked to check the students' temperature every morning; and those in Guangzhou even postponed exams. Upon the suggestion of the inspection team by the State Administration for Tourism, all group tours were terminated until the end of May. The provincial price bureau stipulated stiff fines for hikers of medical drug prices.

In Beijing, the United Working Group for Preventing and Curing ATP, headed by Liu Qi, had a deputy director who was from the military. Thus SARS management incorporated the military system, including its hospitals. Some 1,200 military medical workers were sent to the newly built Xiaotangshan Hospital. Another two hospitals were also used as primary sites to house SARS patients. On April 17, Beijing designated six hospitals for SARS treatment. In the following days, it designated another 11. By May 7, Beijing's capabilities to house and treat SARS in designated hospitals had dramatically improved. In addition, Beijing also established 63 hospitals for treating patients with fevers. These measures helped reduce infections within the hospitals and communities.[23]

Mass Mobilization at All Levels

After the Politburo Standing Committee decided to make SARS a national task, it reverted to its conventional political weapon — campaigns. Campaigns were launched not only at the national bureaucracy, but were also ordered to take place at all local levels. Again, through the center's control and appointment of all cadres, this order of campaign was quickly carried out.

[23] "Behind the reduction of ATP epidemic in Beijing", posted at http://www.chinesenewsnet.com on 13 May 2003, accessed on the same day.

The typical operational mode of campaigns is as follows. Leaders at all levels take personal command of the outstanding task, take personal responsibilities for the outcome, and coordinate activities of various agencies under their jurisdiction, introduce and enforce necessary measures. The media starts to give extensive coverage of the campaign, installing officials and populace with a sense of urgency and driving them into action. Governmental agencies, social institutions, and state economic entities are ordered to take corresponding action. In the case of SARS, even non-state enterprises felt the pressure and would take some, if not all, of the measures prescribed by the state.

As a result of campaign, all localities down to the village level were mobilized. Out of concern of spread of the deadly disease in their localities and to avoid being penalized for the spread of the disease; local leaders usually took up the measures ordered by the Politburo — coordinating local SARS management, finding out, quarantining, and treating in a timely manner SARS patients and suspect cases, taking precautionary measures to avoid the import of the disease from outside, procuring medical equipment and drugs, providing assistance to poor patients, and disclosing epidemic statistics. Some, especially in places with inadequate medical facilities, even took strong-arm measures. Some villages and townships prohibited outsiders and persons who worked in the epidemic areas (such as Guangdong and Beijing) from visiting. A city even went overboard in sabotaging a highway link with Beijing to prevent people from entering the city. The over-zealous cadre responsible for the act was disciplined.

As a precautionary measure, all schools in Beijing were closed for two weeks in the late April and early May. A number of universities were cordoned off and outside visitors were prevented from entering. Many residential communities sanitized themselves. In the outskirts of Beijing, villages installed guards to bar the entry of outsiders.

Conclusion

In the early months, SARS management was hampered by structural flaws in central-local arrangement. Although fully aware of the seriousness of the disease, local leaders and the health leaders under-reported the information to their superiors, and hid it from the public. They did so out of concerns with their own careers. The center overemphasized economic growth in promoting local cadres. As a result, national leaders might have overlooked the danger posed by the disease. Furthermore, provinces lacked the formal authority to order provincial health, tourism, railway, and transportation departments to take stern actions to restrain SARS. They had to consult national offices of these departments before taking any formal measure. However, provincial leaders did have the informal authority to order these local departments. Finally, communication between localities and between public health institutions across the provinces, in the same province, and even in the same city was poor and seriously inadequate. This led to a high infection rate among medical workers. SARS also spread throughout Guangdong and even to Hong Kong, Singapore and Canada.

After mid April, changes in national policies injected new dynamics in central-local interaction and led to effective local management. The center used its control of cadres to force them to take action. It launched a campaign at the national level and compelled all localities to follow suit. It also took the lead in coordinating SARS management. National ministries separately or jointly formulated policies, urging their local branches to take measures to prevent and treat the spread of SARS. On April 17, the Politburo Standing Committee urged all ministries and localities to launch a campaign against SARS. On April 20, the center fired two senior officials for their SARS mismanagement, goading all officials on taking its call for action seriously. It formed a national command center for SARS management and provided a special fund for it. The result was an immediate outburst of energy from the central down to the grassroots levels, detecting, isolating and treating SARS patients, publicizing statistics and calls for treatments, sanitizing public places, and public avoiding risky areas and persons. Guangdong and Beijing were among these mobilized localities. Very soon, SARS was contained in Guangdong, and later on in Beijing and other localities.

On the whole, China's central-local arrangements still suffer from information asymmetries in favor of lower-level officials rather than the higher-level ones and in favor of the state rather than the people. After SARS, the center might try to evaluate local cadres more comprehensively. A lack of formal coordinating authority within a province may still exist. These drawbacks will continue to haunt the Chinese state. On the other hand, the state has several weapons at reserve — dismissal and appointment of local cadres, mass campaign, and national role in coordinating activities. They are indispensable for the state to deal with major crises. However, without overcoming the above drawbacks, a serious problem may develop into a crisis, and the state may have to resort to the costly last resorts of disciplining cadres, taking a personal lead in coordination, and launching mass campaigns.

REFERENCES

Gore, Lance. 1998. *Market Communism: The Institutional Foundation of China's Post-Mao Hyper-Growth*. Hong Kong: Oxford University Press.

Huang, Yasheng. 1996. *Inflation and Investment Controls in China: The Political Economy of Central-Local Relations during the Reform Era*. New York: Cambridge University Press.

Lieberthal, Kenneth. 1992. "Introduction," in David Lampton and Kenneth Lieberthal, eds. *Bureaucracy, Politics, and Decision Making in Post-Mao China*. Berkeley: University of California Press.

Lieberthal, Kenneth. 1995. *Governing China: From Revolution through Reform*. New York: W. W. Norton.

Lieberthal, Kennen and Michel Oksenberg. 1988. *Policy Making in China: Leaders, Structures, and Processes*. Princeton, New Jersey: Princeton University Press.

Ma, Rong. 2003. "Employment: Paying attention to difficult groups amidst challenges", in Ru Xin, Lu Xueyi, and Li Peilin, eds. *2003: Analyses and Predictions of China's Social Situation (2003 Nian: Zhongguo Shehui Xingshi Fenxi Yu Yuce)*. Beijing: Shehui Kexue Wenxian Chubanshe, pp. 35–44.

Stevenson-Yang, Anne. 2003. "The absent-minded reform of China's media", in David M. Finkelstein and Maryanne Kivlehan, eds. *China's Leadership in the 21st Century: The Rise of the Fourth Generation*. Armonk, NY: M.E. Sharpe, pp. 223–248.

Chapter 4

SARS and the Rule of Law in China

Zou Keyuan

Introduction

People may feel curious about the title and wonder whether there is any connection between severe acute respiratory syndrome (SARS) and the rule of law. Superficially, SARS is a fatal epidemic that once haunted and will possibly continue to haunt Asia and the rest of the world while the rule of law mainly concerns development and improvement of a legal system so as to safeguard a country's stability and prosperity as well as individual freedom and rights. The two are irrelevant *prima facie*. However, SARS has triggered a *de facto* revolution in Chinese politics and society in many aspects. It inevitably affects China's ongoing legal reform towards the rule of law as China pledged in its 1999 Constitution Amendment, and forces the Chinese leadership to consider the important role of the law in realizing good governance. Although there is no universally accepted definition of the rule of law, this paper regards it as a process of legal capacity-building and accountability and from the SARS event it can be seen how this process goes, to what extent law *per se* has played its role in the anti-SARS campaign, and what are the legal implications therefrom for the on-going Chinese legal reform.

The Implementation Dilemma

SARS originated in Guangdong Province, China. It was reported that the first SARS case was discovered there as early as November 2002.

China was blamed for the spread of SARS to the rest of the world by its mismanagement at the early period of the outbreak. One of the reasons behind the mismanagement is apparently the failure of the relevant Chinese law enforcement.

China enacted its Law on Prevention and Control of Infectious Diseases in 1989.[1] The Law makes specific stipulations on related principles and policies of the central government about epidemic prevention and treatment. It also lists obligations and urgent measures bestowed on governments of various levels and on medical and public health departments, as well as individuals' rights and duties for the prevention and treatment of infectious diseases. It contains seven chapters and 41 clauses. Infectious diseases are accordingly divided into three categories: infectious diseases (a) including plague and cholera; infectious diseases (b) including 22 diseases such as AIDS, dengue fever, malaria; and infectious diseases (c) including 11 diseases such as tuberculosis, schistosomiasis, and leprosy. In addition, the number of the listed (statutory) diseases may be increased or decreased under different circumstances. According to the Law, governments at all levels have the responsibility to prepare and implement plans for the prevention of infectious diseases. Health departments at all levels should monitor and administer the work of disease prevention and control. Persons in charge and personnel working on disease prevention and control should not conceal actual information or lie or incite to conceal actual information or lie (Article 22). When there is an outbreak of infectious disease, the government in the locality should immediately prevent and cut off the spreading channels. If necessary, the local government, approved by the higher level government, may adopt emergency measures including the suspension of markets, assemblies, plays in cinemas and theaters and other gatherings; suspension of school, work and business operations; temporary requisition of houses and vehicles; and closure of public drinking water source which has been polluted by the infectious virus; and declaration of the affected area as epidemic infected area.

The Law also provides for a reporting system, stipulating that anyone who has found a patient or suspected patient should report to the nearest

[1] Text is available at http://www.moh.gov.cn/wsflfg/fl/200205140007.htm, accessed on 30 Jul 2003.

health organ immediately. Any responsible person in hospitals or other medical organs should report to the local health department, then the local health department report to the local government and the higher level health department and finally to the Ministry of Health.[2] However, the Law does not provide the time limit for the reporting, which can be regarded as a shortcoming in the Law and reporting may be delayed in some circumstances. This loophole was later remedied in the 1991 Implementing Measures.

Social responsibility is imposed on every person living in China. The Law provides that "all units and individuals within the territory of the People's Republic of China must receive questioning, examination, investigation and preventive and control measures about relevant infectious diseases from medical and healthcare organs and sanitation and anti-epidemic organs, and have the right to report and complain any conduct in violation of this Law".[3] Any person who is infected or suspected to be infected should be quarantined for treatment. Refusal for quarantine and treatment or escape from quarantine and treatment is subject to compulsory measures by the treatment unit with the assistance from the police (Article 24). As for the liability, the Law provides administrative punishment, and fines are levied. Criminal liability can also be imposed in certain circumstances such as spreading of infectious diseases under Category A, or spreading of infectious virus and causing serious consequences, or dereliction causing serious consequences.[4]

For the purpose of implementing the 1989 Law, the Ministry of Health issued the Implementing Measures for the Law on Prevention and Control of Infectious Diseases in December 1991.[5] The Measures also divide infectious diseases into three categories, but what is different from the 1989 Law is that the division in the Measures is made according to the nature of germs and viruses rather than diseases so that the viruses of AIDS and smallpox are listed under Category A in addition to germs of

[2] See Article 21 of the 1989 Law.

[3] Article 7 of the 1989 Law.

[4] See Articles 35–39 of the 1989 Law.

[5] Text is available at http://www.moh.gov.cn/wsflfg/fg/200208150010.htm, accessed on 2 Aug 2003.

plague and cholera.[6] Such division may in practice cause confusion with the ones under the 1989 Law, though different wordings are used. It can be interpreted that the 1991 Measures expanded the number of the diseases in Category A of the 1989 Law.

Patients suffering from most of the infectious diseases should be quarantined for treatment. Work units employing more than 200 floating people should report to the health department of the local government and implement hygiene measures as required to prevent and control infectious diseases (Article 20). Water, goods, or excrement polluted by diseases such as typhoid, bacillary dysentery, and hepatitis should be strictly treated. The responsible epidemic reporters are personnel working in hospitals and disease control centers. They should report the diseases of plague, cholera, lung anthrax or AIDS to the local health department with a fastest communicating means no later than 6 hours in towns and 12 hours in countryside from the first discovery of the disease (Article 35). The epidemic situation in the military is to be reported to the State Council by the military health department in accordance with relevant regulations (Article 39). The emergency measures under Article 25 of the 1989 Law can be lifted based on the following conditions: (1) patients are completely healed; (2) polluted goods and surroundings have been disinfected; and (3) no discovery of new patients after the longest incubation period of a disease (Article 54).

The Implementing Measures also contain some provisions on liability including administrative punishment and fines for those who have violated the relevant laws and regulations. In particular, the Measures provide that no responsible person should conceal or delay the reporting, otherwise he is subject to administrative punishment. Nevertheless, in comparison with the new regulations, the liability provisions in both the 1989 Law and the 1991 Measures are very light, and mainly limited to administrative punishment and monetary fines.

The 1989 Law and related measures should have applied to the SARS case from the very beginning when SARS emerged since they were designed to combat infectious diseases. It should be pointed out that though SARS was a new disease beyond human knowledge and its initial

[6] See Article 16 of the 1991 Implementing Measures.

symptoms looked like flu, even if it was regarded and treated as a kind of flu at the beginning, it should be governed by the 1989 Law which lists "flu" under Category C of infectious diseases.[7] Unfortunately, the Law was forgotten and/or ignored at that time. It was mentioned only once at a press conference by a high-rank official from the government health department, blindly saying that the Law was not applicable because SARS was not listed therein.[8] One official explanation for the ignorance of the 1989 Law was that in recent years there had been no wide spread of infectious diseases in China.[9] Only until April 2003 did China realize the importance of the Law.

On April 8, 2003, the Ministry of Health, under the approval of the State Council, put the SARS under the scope of statutory infectious diseases in accordance with the 1989 Law. It is, however, unclear whether SARS is defined as a disease in Category A or B or C. It is assumed that since SARS was declared by the Ministry of Health, it should not be in Category A.

Since then, the Law had begun to display its effect in the anti-SARS campaign. On April 30, a public announcement was made jointly by the Publicity Department of the Central Committee of the Chinese Communist Party (CCP), Ministry of Justice and Ministry of Health that the whole country should keep the fight against SARS in line with the 1989 Law.[10] According to the announcement, the 1989 Law was "of great significance in protecting people's health and in ensuring the prevention and treatment of SARS".[11] Correspondent measures were accordingly taken to set up quarantine zones in affected areas and to activate the system of reporting and publicizing SARS cases. Information on SARS had been given to the public daily since April 20, 2003 (instead of the former

[7] See Article 3 of the 1989 Law.

[8] See Yu Zeyuan. "Health Minister: Epidemic in China has been controlled", *Lianhe Zaobao* (in Chinese), 4 Apr 2003.

[9] See "Zhang Chunsheng thinks more time is needed to improve the anti-infectious diseases law", at http://www.people.com.cn/GB/shehui/1060/1944447.html, accessed 17 Jul 2003.

[10] Text is available in *Legal Daily* (in Chinese), 1 May 2003.

[11] "Law highlighted in fight against SARS in China", *Xinhua News Agency*, 1 May 2003.

practice of every five days). In addition, China punished law-breakers and sacked derelict government officials. Yet this belated legal response from the Chinese government has, at least partly, caused thousands of more SARS victims within and outside China.

NEW REGULATIONS

Significantly, following the announcement, China enacted new regulations on public health emergencies in May 2003, the first of its kind in China.[12] The Regulations aim to establish a prompt and effective emergency response mechanism and enhance the government's ability of handling public health emergencies such as SARS. Public health emergency is defined as serious infectious diseases, massive unknown diseases, serious food or vocational poisoning, which suddenly happen and cause or possibly cause serious damage to public health, and others which seriously affect public health.[13]

The Regulations establish the monitoring, early warning and reporting systems. Upon the emergency happening, the State Council should establish a national command headquarter, composing relevant departments from the government and from the army. Governments at the county level and above should establish and improve the monitoring and warning system.[14] As for the reporting system, it is required that provincial governments should report emergencies to the Ministry of Health within an hour upon the receipt of emergency reports, and monitoring and medical institutions should report the emergencies to the county level health department within two hours.[15] It also provides that any individual or organization has the right to report emergencies and enjoys the right to accuse governments of not performing their duties according to law. Contingency plans should be prepared both at the central and provincial levels. Governments and officials will be held responsible for hiding or delaying emergency information or giving false information.

[12] Text is available in *People's Daily* (in Chinese), 13 May 2003, p. 8.

[13] Article 2 of the 2003 Regulations.

[14] See Article 14 of the 2003 Regulations.

[15] See Article 20 of the 2003 Regulations.

The Regulations establish the emergency information publicizing system as well. During the SARS period, the information on SARS was publicized every day.

Legal liabilities will be imposed if the conduct of relevant persons is deemed to have broken the law. The Regulations set forth five types of punishment on government officials if they have concealed or delayed the reporting or lied; have failed to accomplish the tasks of producing, supplying or transporting the materials which are needed for the emergencies; have failed to cooperate or hampered or intervened investigations; dereliction; failed to follow the instructions for handling emergencies; and failed to control the spreading of infectious diseases.[16] In addition, any entity or person who has failed to abide by the Regulations will be punished as well. It is particularly provided that during the emergency period, those who spread rumors, raise prices, cheat customers, and disturb social and market order, will be punished.

The new regulations can be regarded as an extension and update of the 1989 Law since it elaborates on and further specializes the relevant provisions in that Law. For example, Article 30 of the 2003 Regulations provides the procedure of declaring statutory infectious diseases, which follows the relevant stipulations in the 1989 Law. Furthermore, the Regulations contain modern "rule of law" elements, such as a responsible reporting system, public participation and punishment of delinquent officials. In comparison, the 1989 Law was enacted during the time when China still followed the planned economy policy and exercised rigid political control such that quite a number of its clauses need an update. It is acknowledged that China had previously developed laws to deal with emergencies like earthquakes and floods, but the country's public health system was not well prepared for the SARS epidemic. The new regulations are designed to overcome the weaknesses of the public health system to fight against SARS by making full use of the law and fill a gap in the Chinese legal system.[17] Even Chinese Premier Wen Jiabao considered the newly enacted regulations on public health emergencies a powerful

[16] See Articles 45–50 of the 2003 Regulations.

[17] See "China improves legal system to cope with public health emergencies", *Xinhua News Agency*, 14 May 2003.

weapon to defeat SARS and a major step towards ensuring China handles health crises. Wen requested local governments above county level to establish disease prevention and control centers and to set up a contingency troop of medical workers to handle emergencies in public health according to law.[18] Song Ruilin, vice-director of the Department of Science, Education, Culture and Health in the Legislative Affairs Office of the State Council, which was a major drafter of the Regulations, expressed that the Regulations represent a legislative breakthrough in requiring governments at all levels to report crisis information without delay. A public health emergency is a social issue that has a great impact on the country. "That is why the Regulations put a heavy responsibility on governments to enhance management and unified command".[19]

Instead of using vague terms such as "timely" and "immediately", the Regulations have set a time limit for governments to report crises, highlighting the need for quick response.

The Regulations say provincial governments must report emergencies to State public health authorities within an hour of receiving reports of an emergency. According to Song, "the clear time limit has actually nailed down the responsibility of governments and serves as a benchmark for telling whether officials have delayed information". Time means life in a public health emergency so that it is vital to have a specific time limit for reporting.[20]

Meanwhile, concerns also arise regarding the enforcement of the new regulations. The criminal liability stipulated in the Regulations is an example. Although the Regulations do not expressly provide exact criminal punishment, the explanation on the Regulations from the relevant Chinese authorities indicated that the punishment could be as severe as death penalty imposed on a law-breaker, though China's practice shows no sign of using death penalty during the anti-SARS campaign. This harshness was criticized not only by human rights activists, but also by the World Health Organization and other governments. Judging by this example, there is a sufficient reason to believe that China's current way

[18] "Law to help better control epidemic — Premier", *China Daily*, 16 May 2003.
[19] See "Law to help better control epidemic — Premier", *China Daily*, 16 May 2003.
[20] "Law to help better control epidemic — Premier", *China Daily*, 16 May 2003.

toward the rule of law is still premature and the use of law as a pure instrument of government control contradicts the spirit of the rule of law.

Administration by Law

In the post-WTO era, governments at all levels in China have to change their means of management from the previously administrative one to the current legal one. Law will become more and more important in government management. Administration by law (*yi fa xing zheng*) becomes a popular slogan used by governments at all level. Law is designed to limit government power, to establish adequate administrative procedures and to formulate the conception of responsible governance.

Limit of government power is manifested in the recent developments of administrative law in China. Administrative law refers to the laws and regulations governing the administrative relations between the governmental organs and ordinary citizens.[21] During the last two decades and more, the development of administrative law in China can be divided into two periods, before and after 1989 when the Law of Administrative Procedure was enacted and implemented.[22] In the first period, there were two important laws which came into being: the 1982 Law on Civil Procedure (provisional) and the 1987 Regulations on the Punishment in Public Security Management. They, in particular the provisions therein relating to administrative procedure, provided a basis for the emergence of administrative law.

The milestone in the development of administrative law in China is the promulgation of the Law on Administrative Procedure in 1989. It is said that the establishment of the legal regime of administrative procedure means the establishment of "a democratic system".[23] This law, for the first time, set the detailed standards to define which are legal or illegal administrative activities. The People's Court has the right to repeal the illegal administrative activities. The 1994 State Compensation Law

[21] See Xu Hua & Yu Jie, eds. 1998. *China's 20 Years Construction of Legal System* (in Chinese). Zhengzhou: Zongzhou Old Document Publishing House, p. 118.

[22] See Ying Songnian. 1998. "Developments of the Chinese Administrative Law", *Zengfa Luntan* (Journal of China University of Political Science and Law), No. 5, p. 18.

[23] Ying, *ibid.*, p. 19.

is a big supplement to the Law on Administrative Procedure. It has developed the administrative procedure system by establishing a compensation system. According to a Chinese legal scholar, the legal elements embodied in the above two laws are advanced, such as proof by the defence, time limit, compulsory enforcement in the Law on Administrative Procedure, and liability principle of compensation for illegal activities, and compensation liability for damages resulting from factual acts.[24]

Another important development in administrative law is the 1996 Law on Administrative Punishment. It governs the administrative activities which impose punishment upon violations. From this perspective, it is different from the laws on administrative procedure or on State compensation. It sets forth several principles: (1) no punishment shall be ever imposed when there is no express stipulation for such punishment; (2) the right to prescribe in terms of punishment for personal rights or property rights only belongs to law; and (3) the procedure for administrative punishment is for the first time detailed in the law, particularly the hearing system which is quite new in China. For these reasons, it can be said that it is one of the important milestones for the rule of law in China.[25] After this law, other major laws were also enacted in this respect, including the Law on Administrative Review Procedure (adopted in April 1999), and the Law on Administrative Licensing (passed in August 2003).[26]

The Law on Administrative Licensing defines "administrative licensing" as the conduct of an administrative organ to examine and approve a certain specified activity which has applied for.[27] Public health and ecological environmental protection are two main areas which require administrative licensing. Any regulation on administrative licensing should be publicized; otherwise they cannot become the basis to grant an administrative license.[28] A citizen, legal person or organization enjoys the

[24] Ying, *ibid.*, p. 19. A case on State compensation was reported. Peng Jie, a lawyer who was wrongly prosecuted and judged, got the compensation as well as the apology. See "Peng Jie got state compensation according to the law", *Legal Daily* (in Chinese), 7 Nov 1998.

[25] See Ying, "Developments of the Chinese Administrative Law", pp. 19–20.

[26] Text is available in *People's Daily* (in Chinese), 28 Aug 2003, p. 13. It will come into force from 1 Jul 2004.

[27] Article 2 of the Administrative Licensing Law.

[28] Article 5 of the Administrative Licensing Law.

right to presentation and explanation, the right to apply for administrative review or launch an administrative litigation. The new law explicitly forbids government agencies from empowering themselves with the right to grant permits or collecting fees not required by law. Through the implementation of the Law, the amount of administrative licensing will be greatly reduced and departments under the State Council will no longer have the right to determine whether a certain economic activity needs an administrative permit. While the Law has been hailed as "a great help in China's efforts to build a market economy and check corruption",[29] its implementation will meet a series of challenges. First, the Law only provides general principles which result in ambiguities and would turn the law into an un-enforceable dilemma in practice. Second, the advanced legal spirit embodied in the Law may not be endorsed by the government and its officials who have such administrative power in hand for a long time and "the implementation of the Law will inevitably conflict with vested interests".[30] Nevertheless, by the time when the administrative licensing law was adopted, a relative administrative law had been formulated to curb the administrative power and to prevent power abuse as well as official corruption. It is reported that during the SARS period, many officials were sacked due to their incompetence. For example, 207 cadres in Hunan Province and 223 in Anhui Province were punished by Party disciplines and/or state laws.[31]

The development of administrative law is also linked to the WTO requirements. On the one hand, governments at all levels should administer by law and on the other hand they should follow the transparency principle set forth by the WTO law. The publicizing requirement stipulated in the Administrative Licensing Law is a typical example. In addition, after the WTO entry, China is unable to continue using large amount of normative internal documents to govern the society. Instead, the government documents, when needed and in line with the WTO regulations, should be reflected in the form of laws and regulations. For that

[29] "New law to help streamline licensing", *China Daily*, 1 Sept 2003.

[30] "Commentary: Law keeps government in check", *China Daily*, 6 Sept 2003.

[31] See Chen Feng. "Official sacking storm should pay regard to the legitimate procedure", in http://www.iolaw.org.cn/feidian/shownews.asp?id=1086, accessed on 26 Jul 2003.

purpose, during the SARS period, various government departments passed large amount of administrative regulations ranging from public health, transportation, protection of wildlife and environment to prices, etc. (see Table 1).

Table 1. Selected Administrative Regulations and Measures Relating to SARS

- Notice on Tax Deduction Preferential Policy for Anti-SARS Donations by Ministry of Finance and Taxation Bureau (29/04/2003)
- Emergent Notice on Vaccination for Diseases Control by Ministry of Health (29/04/2003)
- Management Rules for Reporting on National Disasters and Public Health Emergencies by Ministry of Health (04/04/2003)
- Conditions on National Non-infected Areas by Ministry of Health (08/07/2002)
- Measures on Prevention, Treatment and Management of SARS by Ministry of Health (13/05/2003)
- Notice on Training of Medical Personnel for Prevention and Treatment of Infectious Diseases by Ministry of Health (01/07/2003)
- Diagnostical Standards for SARS and TB Verification by Ministry of Health (09/05/2003)
- Verification Standards for SARS Close Contacted Persons by Ministry of Health (08/05/2003)
- New Guidelines for SARS Control in Hospitals by Ministry of Health (04/05/2003)
- Standards for SARS Clinical Diagnosis, Treatment and Discharge by Ministry of Health (03/05/2003)
- Principles for Design and Construction of Hospitals for SARS Patients by Ministries of Health and Construction (14/05/2003)
- Guideline Principles for SARS Disinfection in Public Places by Ministry of Health (07/05/2003)
- Urgent Circular on Further Strengthening the Prevention and Control of SARS by Ministry of Communications (25/04/2003)
- Contingent Plan for Road and Waterway Transport During SARS Period by Ministry of Communications (29/04/2003)
- Circular on Change of Foreign Currencies by Foreign Students Who Withdrew from Schools in China by Bureau of Foreign Exchange Management (29/04/2003)
- Interpretation on Applying Certain Laws for Criminal Cases Resulting from Hampering the Prevention and Control of Suddenly Emerged Infectious Diseases by the Supreme Court and the Supreme Procuratorate (15/05/2003)

Source: Prepared by the author.

The Ministry of Health played a most active role in this respect. It adopted a specific regulation on SARS — Measures on SARS Prevention, Treatment and Management in May 2003.[32] It is based on the 1989 Law and the 2003 Regulations, but unlike them, it is specifically designed to combat SARS. According to it, SARS is a statutory infectious disease under the 1989 Law (Article 2). It also issued a Notice of training health personnel on how to prevent and control infectious diseases in July 2003.[33] Health organs should launch two kinds of training programs: long-term and urgent, and the urgent training programs should be completed by October 15, 2003. Other government departments adopted administrative rules within their jurisdictional competence.

In addition, local legislations also play an important role (see Table 2). For example, Guangdong Province began to improve its system of treating infectious disease patients by adopting the Guidelines for the Construction of the System of Infectious Diseases Patients Treatment in August 2003. Accordingly, the province has planned to spend one year and a half to establish such a system covering the whole province including urban and rural areas.[34] Meanwhile, responsible treatment system in hospitals has been established as well.[35] Shanghai's People's Congress Standing Committee adopted the Decision on Strengthening the Prevention and Control of SARS in May 2003.[36] The Regulations on Management of Urban Environment was also amended. Accordingly, the fines on illegal spitting were raised from 50 RMB to 200 RMB from the

[32] Text is available at http://www.10thnpc.org.cn/chinese/PI-c/329479.htm, accessed on 21 Jul 2003.

[33] Text is available at http://www.moh.gov.cn/kjjy/gzdt/yxjy/1200307080012.htm, accessed on 2 Aug 2003.

[34] See "Guangdong Province began to improve its system of infectious disease patients treatment", at http://www.hsm.com.cn/node2/node116/node275/node276/userobject6ai113433.html, accessed on 8 Aug 2003.

[35] See "Doctors who delay SARS report may be prosecuted", *Mingpao* (in Chinese), 29 Oct 2003.

[36] See "Shanghai People's Congress for the first time launches urgent legislation to curb SARS", 13 May 2003, at http://www.npcnews.com.cn/gb/special/calss000000039/1/hwz235877.htm, accessed on 17 Jul 2003.

Table 2. Selected Local Laws and Regulations Relating to SARS

- Implementing Measures concerning the Regulations on Public Health Emergencies by Hainan Province (2003)
- Decision on Prevention and Control of Spreading of SARS by Hainan Province (2003)
- Implementing Measures concerning the Regulations on Public Health Emergencies by Hunan Province (2003)
- Measures concerning Public Health Emergencies by Nanjing City (2003)
- Measures concerning Public Health Emergencies by Shandong Province (03/06/2003)
- Regulations on Patriotic Health (amended) by Shanxi Province (29/05/2003)
- Notice on Taking Quarantine Measures in SARS-Affected Areas by Beijing Municipality (20/04/2003)
- Certain Measures on SARS Prevention and Control by Beijing Municipality (28/05/2003)
- Patriotic Health Regulations by Guangdong Province (25/07/2003)
- Certain Provisions on Prohibition of Eating Wild Animals by Shenzhen Special Economic Zone (01/10/2003)

Source: Prepared by the author.

date of April 25, 2003.[37] Though there was no SARS patient in Hainan, this province also took high vigilance and was the second after Shanghai to adopt anti-SARS regulations.[38]

Problems, however, still remain in the administration by law. First, not all officials and/or government departments are used to this new governance method as required. Some still issue internal documents during the SARS period. That is why there is a complaint in China that too many "red dotted documents" (*hongdou wenjian*) are flying over the sky based on the administrative discretion, which would be suspected of abuse of administrative power. For that reason, the role of people's congresses

[37] The fines on spitting on the streets was first put into the local law in 1984. The amount was 0.2 RMB, and in 1988, it was raised to 10 RMB, and in April 2002, to 50 RMB. See "Special legislation in the special period", at http://www.iolaw.org.cn/feidian/shownews.asp?id=1257, accessed on 26 Jul 2003.

[38] See "Hainan People's Congress Standing Committee adopted the decision on SARS spreading", 13 Jun 2003, at http://www.peopledaily.com.cn/GB/14576/14957/1913898.html, accessed on 14 Aug 2003.

should be strengthened and the government power should be endorsed by people's congresses through legislation.[39] In a transitional society like China, such old practices may co-exist for a time with the new practice, but the new one will eventually replace the old one completely.

Second, people question the procedure of declaring SARS as a statutory infectious disease by raising the concern that the declaration was made by the Ministry of Health, but not the State Council. However, it is treated in practice as a disease under Category A of the 1989 Law which provides that the power to add or delete any infectious disease in Category A should belong to the State Council. The date of publicizing is also questionable in accordance with the requirement of administration by law and transparency principle: the date when SARS was designated as a statutory infectious disease was April 8, 2003 through an internal document by the Ministry of Health distributed to its subordinated institutions and medical units, and only until April 14 was it publicized through media.[40] The problem is during this gap of time, the effective control of SARS would be delayed. It is also concerned with the right to information enjoyed by Chinese citizens. As required by the 1989 Law, the Ministry of Health should publicize it timely without delay. Clearly, in the eyes of some, officials in the Ministry did not pay enough attention to this legal requirement. It is remembered that the new government led by Hu Jintao and Wen Jiabao have promised a government more attuned to the people's needs.[41]

SARS AND THE CHINESE COURTS

It is well predicted that the next battlefield on SARS could be the courtroom.[42] Various and numerous cases will emerge from the SARS event.

[39] See Cheng Jie. "Prevention and treatment of SARS needs the exercise of power by people's congresses", at http://www.iolaw.org.cn/feidian/shownews.asp?id=790, accessed on 26 Jul 2003.

[40] See Li Yong and Wu Xiaoliang. "SARS into the law", http://www.iolaw.org.cn/feidian/shownews.asp?id=954, accessed on 26 Jul 2003.

[41] John Pomfret. "China's slow reaction to fast-moving illness, fearing loss of control, Beijing stonewalled", *Washington Post*, 3 Apr 2003, p. A18.

[42] "Courtrooms may become next SARS battleground", *China Daily*, 26 May 2003.

They may include criminal, civil as well as administrative cases. The courts have already been handling such cases since the SARS outbreak.

Criminal Cases

The Supreme Court and the Supreme Procuratorate jointly issued the judicial interpretation on applying certain laws for criminal cases resulting from the hampering of prevention and control of suddenly emerged infectious diseases on May 15, 2003. According to it, intentional spreading of infectious diseases is a crime of endangering public security and should be punished as such. The degree of punishment could be from ten years of imprisonment to death penalty. SARS patients or suspected patients who refuse to be quarantined or receive treatment and spread the epidemic by fault will be punished with three to ten years of imprisonment. According to a Beijing legislation, fines can also be imposed for escapees from 5,000 RMB to 20,000 RMB.[43]

Based on the above interpretation, the Supreme Procuratorate requested procuratorates at all levels to investigate and handle six types of dereliction cases including negligence or abuse of power (opposable to government officials); delay or non-performance of duties (opposable to personnel in medical organs); dereliction (opposable to personnel working in education, railway, transport, civil aviation, tourism); irresponsibility (opposable to personnel working in quarantine departments); corruption and dereliction (opposable to personnel working in industry and commerce administration, medicine supervisory administration and management of prices); and dereliction (opposable to personnel working in governments and public security).[44] The Criminal Law provides that jail terms of less than three years will be imposed on any government employee who conducts a serious dereliction of duty. The Beijing People's

[43] "Beijing impose fines up to 20,000 on those escape from SARS prevention and control", 30 May 2003, at http://www.people.com.cn/GB/shehui/43/20030530/1004403.html, accessed on 17 Jul 2003.

[44] See "Supreme Procuratorate requests to target six dereliction cases during the SARS period", *Procuratorate Daily* (in Chinese), 21 May 2003, at http://www.10thnpc.org.cn/chinese/zhuanti/feidian/333159.htm, accessed on 21 Jul 2003.

Procuratorate issued a notice in May 2003 saying that governments and its officials who suppress information about SARS will be prosecuted. But it is not clear whether officials who were released from service due to negligence of duty in April, like former Mayor Meng Xuenong of Beijing, will be hit with legal action. Following the request by the Supreme Procuratorate, the Beijing Procuratorate will investigate six different types of SARS-related dereliction of duty and will include the investigation of officials and medical workers.[45] However, according to an authoritative source, concealing or delaying the reporting before the enforcement of the national measures against SARS will be immune from criminal punishment.[46]

In July 2003, the Supreme Court published a judicial decision on a case of blackmail by using SARS. Mao Fangjun, a farmer in Zhejiang Province took the advantage of the people's fear of SARS and made a plot with another farmer Wang Beihu in late April 2003. In early May, Mao sent blackmail letters to two persons respectively, asking them each to transfer 50,000 RMB to his bank account, otherwise, he would transfer SARS to them. The two persons reported to the police and the suspects were arrested on 5 May with no success of extortion. The court in Fenghua, Zhejiang Province sentenced Mao to five years and Wang to two years of imprisonment under the crime of extortion based on Article 274 of the Criminal Code.[47]

Civil Cases

Civil cases are more complicated than criminal cases since they involve various legal subject-matters ranging from insurance claims to medical compensation. As reported, health authorities, medical workers, hospitals and patients were likely to be involved in legal wrangling over the sharp

[45] "Courtrooms may become next SARS battleground", *China Daily*, 26 May 2003.

[46] See "Two highs experts: No criminal liability for concealing epidemic information before the state took action", 16 May 2003, at http://www.10thnpc.org.cn/chinese/law/331071.htm, accessed on 21 Jul 2003.

[47] See "Supreme Court published a judicial decision on the case of blackmailing", at http://www.iolaw.org.cn/feidian/shownews.asp?id=880, accessed on 26 Jul 2003.

SARS infection rate in Beijing hospitals during the initial outbreak of the epidemic. However, some hospitals were likely to be exempt from legal responsibility because of the complicated and unpredicted nature of the previously unknown killer disease. Zhao Xiaojun, an official with the Beijing People's Procuratorate, said that it would not bring any action against hospitals where cross-infection occurred in March and early April.[48] In fact the Beijing Xicheng District Health Bureau received a dozen complaints against hospitals in May 2003. According to one authoritative source, "[s]ome SARS patients, who were infected in hospitals due to the lack of sufficient isolation measures, and their family members have begun to prepare to prosecute for faulty medical treatment".[49] Zhang Xiaolin, a standing committee member of the Beijing Municipal Committee of the Chinese Peasants' and Workers' Democratic Party, said the government would have to interpret whether cross infection was considered medical malpractice. According to the current procedure for handling medical malpractice, "unpredicted and urgent" cases could be exempt from punishment. However, according to him, it is still difficult to judge at present according to the procedure as it does not further illustrate what are unpredicted and urgent.[50]

There is a case concerning a university professor who was allegedly infected with SARS while at Renmin Hospital early April. Whereas the Beijing Municipal Center for Disease Control and Prevention and the hospital should take responsibility for his infection, he was not prepared to sue the two organizations because the possibility of winning the case was minimal due to the ambiguity in the relevant laws.[51]

The legal issue as to whether SARS could constitute *force majeure* is extensively discussed in China. There is a case in Nanjing which ruled that SARS did not constitute *force majeure*. On November 15, 2002, Mr. Zhang (plaintiff) signed a contract with the Nanjing Jaguar Food Limited (the defendant) to run a restaurant under that company to provide food and drink services for tourist groups from January 1, 2003. In April 2003,

[48] "Courtrooms may become next SARS battleground", *China Daily*, 26 May 2003.
[49] "Courtrooms may become next SARS battleground", *China Daily*, 26 May 2003.
[50] "Courtrooms may become next SARS battleground", *China Daily*, 26 May 2003.
[51] "Courtrooms may become next SARS battleground", *China Daily*, 26 May 2003.

because of SARS, the restaurant was trapped in dire straits. Mr. Zhang was unable to continue his performance for the contract and asked to terminate it for the reason of *force majeure*. No result was reached after several rounds of negotiations between the plaintiff and the defendant. The dispute then was brought to the court. The court held that the sudden change of the business environment caused by SARS and the subsequent loss by the change of circumstances should not be borne unilaterally, and the loss should be divided between the two sides. As a result, the contract was terminated with the compensation to the defendant. [52] The court decision indicates that it did not accept the reason of *force majeure* resulting from SARS as a sufficient excuse to release contractual duties. However, the court acknowledged that SARS could be a factor causing fundamental change of circumstances under which contracts could be terminated.

Administrative Cases

So far there is no administrative case available in China, but it does not mean that such cases will not emerge in the future. It is reported that in Hong Kong families of SARS victims were prepared to sue the government for compensation due to the mismanagement of the government during the SARS period.[53] The administrative litigation in Hong Kong will encourage the SARS victims in Mainland China to institute similar lawsuits against the Chinese government.

[52] See "First civil case resulting from SARS in Nanjing, SARS not constitute *force majeure*", at http://www.iolaw.org.cn/feidian/shownews.asp?id=1139, accessed on 29 Sept 2003.

[53] See "SARS expert report publicized today, Hong Kong government may face lawsuits from more SARS patients", *Lianhe Zaobao*, 2 Oct 2003, at http://www.zaobao.com.sg/gj/zg007_021003.html, accessed on 2 Oct 2003. It is reported that the victims living in the Amoy Garden have hired lawyers for preparations for the possible lawsuit against the government. See "No punishment for officials, Amoy Garden residents prepared to sue the government", *China Times* (in Chinese), 3 Oct 2003, at http://news.chinatimes.com/Chinatimes/newslist/newslist-content/0,3546,110505+112003100300077,00.html, accessed on 3 Oct 2003.

MEETING INTERNATIONAL STANDARDS

It is emphasized that after the entry into the WTO the Chinese legal system should follow international rules and regulations. Special reference to relevant international standards has become a routine in Chinese legislation. As reflected in the above new legislations, international standards are considered and more specifically the spirit of the rule of law is manifested in such legislations.

The main and specific international law regulating infectious diseases, in particular SARS, is the International Health Regulations (IHR) which was adopted in 1969 and entered into force in 1971.[54] China was one of the original members of WHO and signed the WHO Constitution on July 22, 1946. The seat in WHO was occupied by the representative from the Republic of China (ROC) until 1972 when the People's Republic of China (PRC) notified the WHO Director-General to participate in the WHO activities. This transfer of representation was a result from the transfer of the United Nations seat to China.[55] Accordingly, the PRC notified the WHO in May 1979 of its recognition of the IHR which should legally bind the PRC as from June 1, 1979.[56]

The IHR is a comprehensive body of international health law and contains relevant stipulations concerning the infectious diseases. It contains 107 clauses and 6 appendixes. The main purpose of the IHR is to prevent and control infectious diseases which are defined in the Regulations as "quarantinable diseases" including cholera, plague, smallpox and yellow fever.[57] WHO member states are obliged to notify WHO of any outbreak of infectious diseases designated above and of any measures they have taken against such diseases. The Regulations require relevant member states to impose measures on health and vaccination for

[54] Text is available in the United Nations Treaty Series website: http://untreaty.un.org (accessed on 2 Aug 2003). Strictly speaking, the IHR was originally adopted in 1951, but at that time its name was the International Sanitary Regulations.

[55] Ironically, ROC still legally presents China in the UN system but all such seats were actually occupied by PRC.

[56] See "List of multilateral treaties China acceded to", at http://www.fmprc.gov.cn/chn/premade/45115/duobian.htm, accessed on 2 Aug 2003.

[57] See Article 1 of the IHR.

travelers, deratting, disinfecting and disinsecting of transport vehicles and health measures at airports and seaports. It defines the terms such as "disinsecting", "epidemic", "health administration", "health authority", "imported case", "infected area", "infected person", "in quarantine" and "isolation".[58] These terms are related to the measures against SARS.

The Regulations have played a positive role in preventing the outbreak and spreading of infectious diseases. However, it has limitations. As realized by the WHO, there are five main shortcomings: limited coverage (only four diseases); dependence on country notification; lack of mechanisms for collaboration; lack of incentives; and lack of risk-specific measures.[59] The proposed revisions accordingly concern ten areas including the reporting system for all public health emergencies of international concern; the need of a focal point in each member country for the IHR renewal process; the need of the country's capacity to quickly report and analyze national disease risks and to determine their potential to spread internationally; the option of making confidential and provisional notifications to the WHO; the use of information other than official notification by the WHO to help identify and control public health emergencies of international concern and the obligation of the member country to respond to requests from the WHO to verify the reliability of such information; the offset of economic losses associated with public health emergencies suggested by the WHO; obligation of the WHO to rapidly assist member States; a transparent process within the WHO to issue recommendations; a non-exhaustive list of key measures; and establishment of a permanent IHR review body.[60] Under the proposed revisions, a member state of the WHO like China bears the obligation to notify the WHO of public health emergencies of international concern; respond to requests for verification of information regarding urgent national risks; control urgent national public health risks that threaten to transmit disease to other member states; provide routine and emergent port of

[58] *Ibid.*

[59] See WHO. "Global crises — Global solutions: Managing public health emergencies of international concern through the revised International Health Regulations", WHO/CDS/CSR/ GAR/2002.4, 2002, p. 3.

[60] *Ibid.*, pp. 5–10.

entry/embarkation inspection and control activities to prevent international disease transmission; and to apply the measures recommended by the WHO during public health emergencies.[61]

The WHO acknowledged that the SARS outbreak provides firm evidence of the urgent need for revising and updating the IHR.[62] The revision of the IHR has been put on the agenda of the World Health Assembly since 1995, but the SARS outbreak obviously has accelerated its process. It was decided during the 56th Assembly that an intergovernmental working group should be established to review and recommend a draft revision of the IHR for consideration by the Health Assembly and urged member states "to establish immediately a national standing task force or equivalent group" so as to provide, together with other missions, resources and cooperation to facilitate the revision progress.[63] It is interesting to note that the revision of the IHR is coincided with the revision of the Chinese Law on infectious diseases. China's involvement in the revision of international regulations can no doubt facilitate the revision of its own law, though it is wondered to what extent China can be able to play its role in such a revision. Active participation in global legislation is China's traditional weak point as illustrated in the negotiations of various world laws.[64]

Apart from IHR, other international standards need also to be considered in the prevention and control of infectious diseases, such as relevant regulations adopted under the auspices of the WHO and rules and norms in the field of international human rights law. They will not be discussed in this paper.

CONCLUDING REMARKS

What lies ahead is the need to revise the 1989 Law which proved inadequate in its enforcement during the anti-SARS campaign. For example,

[61] *Ibid.*, p. 12.

[62] See WHO. "Severe acute respiratory syndrome (SARS): Status of the outbreak and lessons for the immediate future", Geneva, 20 May 2003, p. 7.

[63] See "Revision of the International Health Regulations", WHA56.28, 28 May 2003.

[64] It is remembered that none of any clauses in the 1982 Convention on the Law of the Sea was initiated by China during the Third United Nations Conference on the Law of the Sea during 1973–1982.

the Law does not have any clear provision on whether a hospital has the right to refuse to take in patients of infectious diseases. Such refusal happened during the early SARS period. Second, there is no provision on legal liability imposed on those patients who refuse to be quarantined.[65] It is reported that the revision of the 1989 Law has been put on the legislation agenda in the NPC.[66] Other related laws also need necessary revisions due to the SARS factor. For example, the Law on the Protection of Wildlife, which is linked to the prohibition of eating wild games such as civet cats. It has been also targeted as one of the laws to be revised in the NPC legislation plan.[67]

China openly acknowledged that it had paid "a high price" in the fight against SARS.[68] Part of the price was obviously paid for its low legal consciousness and weak law enforcement. According to Gao Qiang, there are six defects in China's disease prevention and control system, and the slow construction of health law is one of them, which is also reflected in weak law enforcement.[69] Nevertheless, SARS gives China a lesson on how to respect the law and how to effectively enforce the law. At the National Working Conference on SARS Control which was held on July 28, 2003, Hu Jingtao, President of the PRC and Secretary-General of the CCP summarized eight experiences from the anti-SARS campaign and one of them

[65] See "Zhang Chunsheng thinks more time is needed to improve the anti-infectious diseases law", at http://www.people.com.cn/GB/shehui/1060/1944447.html, accessed on 17 Jul 2003.

[66] See "Amendment to the Law on Prevention and Control of Infectious Disease has been urgently listed in the legislation plan", *People's Daily* (overseas edition) (in Chinese), 17 Jun 2003, at http://www.peopledaily.com.cn/GB/14576/14957/1919456.html, accessed on 14 Aug 2003.

[67] See Sun Youhai. "Main revising points of the Wildlife Protection Law", *Legal Daily* (in Chinese), 23 Jul 2003.

[68] See "Speech of Mr. Gao Qiang, Executive Vice Minister, Ministry of Health, People's Republic of China", WHO Global Meeting on SARS, Kuala Lumpur, 17 Jun 2003, at http://www.who.int/csr/sars/conference/june_2003/materials/presentations/qiang/en/print.ht..., accessed on 30 Jul 2003.

[69] See "High rank official in the Chinese Ministry of Health admits six defects in China's disease prevention and control system", 26 Aug 2003, at http://www.hsm.com.cn/node2/node116/node275/node276/userobject6ai116886.html, accessed on 26 Aug 2003.

was the insistence on adopting and applying laws and regulations, governing and administering by law so that law had become a strong safeguard in the victory in the fight of the disease.[70] It proved in practice that the application of the relevant laws and regulations helped to win the anti-SARS battle in China. It is perceived that China will emphasize more on the importance of the law from this experience, and will genuinely reach the realm of the rule of law in the foreseeable future.

On the other hand, it should be realized that SARS is the first severe and readily transmissible new disease to emerge in the 21st century.[71] It is a new challenge not only to China but also to the whole world. The effective combatant against SARS relies on the effort of the whole world community. China's cooperation with other countries, particularly the neighboring countries, is necessary. China has paid attention to foreign experiences in combating SARS and in particular, the American emergency response system has been appreciated since SARS was not widespread in the United States.[72] In this respect, international health law becomes ever more important. The rule of law should be realized everywhere in the world.

[70] "Hu Jingtao summarizes eight insightful points in China's anti-SARS campaign", at http://www.hsm.com.cn/node2/node116/node275/node276/userobject6ai111015.html, accessed on 29 Jul 2003.

[71] See WHO. "Severe acute respiratory syndrome (SARS): Status of the outbreak and lessons for the immediate future", Geneva, 20 May 2003, p. 1.

[72] See Huang Jianshi. "Looking into the emergency response system from the United States where there was no wide spread SARS", *People's Daily* (in Chinese), 26 Sept 2003, p. 14.

Chapter 5

Healthcare Regime Change and the SARS Outbreak in China

GU XIN

The severe acute respiratory syndrome (SARS) is a new disease. A variety of health systems functioning in different countries and regions and with different models were severely hit by this new infectious disease in spring 2002. The SARS epidemic in China, however, broke out against the background of a dramatic health system change. Institutional changes in an ailing and transitional health system partially contributed to the SARS outbreak in the early stage, and hamper disease control later on.

The whole health sector in China is now rapidly moving towards marketization and commercialization. The old system of the public provision of almost all healthcare services and the centralized state control over the sector is being dismantled. Most Chinese healthcare providers are increasingly relying on the service-for-fee mode of operating, and the majority of Chinese patients have to pay their healthcare bills from their own pockets. In brief, accompanying the rapid marketization of the whole sector is the sharp decline in the state's financing role in both public and private healthcare services.

One of the major indicators widely used in health policy studies to examine the state's role in financing healthcare services is the proportion of government spending to the total health expenditure (THE). China's THE, as Figure 1 shows, went up from 1994 onwards in both actual value and percentage of GDP. However, Figure 2 shows that the THE growth was caused largely by the sharp increase in personal spending on health care services. The proportion of both government and corporate spending on healthcare experienced sharp decline over the 1990s.[1] This trend continued until 2002 when the share of governmental spending in THE recorded a slight increase. Government health expenditure as percentage of total health expenditure is widely used as an indicator to measure the state's role in financing healthcare services. In examining this indicator from an internationally comparative perspective, Figure 3 shows that the Chinese government displays only a little bit more commitment to the health sector than the governments in low-income countries.

All of these have resulted in the inadequateness of the Chinese health system to handle public health crisis like the SARS epidemic. The inadequateness is manifested, at least, in three aspects as follows:

1. **The dominance of out-of-pocket healthcare finance,** or by the same token, **the lack of a universal health insurance system**. This led to the situation whereby certain groups of population not covered by any medical insurance schemes were particularly vulnerable to the SARS epidemic.
2. **The commercialization of healthcare providers**. This has resulted in rapid growth of healthcare service costs, and as a result many Chinese patients simply do not seek for healthcare until their sickness becomes severe. The failure of SARS patients to receive timely treatment is an important factor for the spread of the SARS epidemic.
3. **The increasing decline of government spending on public health**. Consequently, a wide range of public health services, in particular those unlikely to produce high revenue to the providers, has been underprovided. Therefore, the whole public health system failed to promptly respond to the crisis.

[1] When examining this issue, normally only a division between public and private health spending is made. In China, however, the health spending is divided into three parts: government, corporate, and individual. A large proportion of spending on publicly run health insurance, which is called "social health insurance" in China *vis-à-vis* "private health insurance", is paid by enterprises and other kinds of organizations. Therefore, most of the corporate spending can be regarded as "public spending".

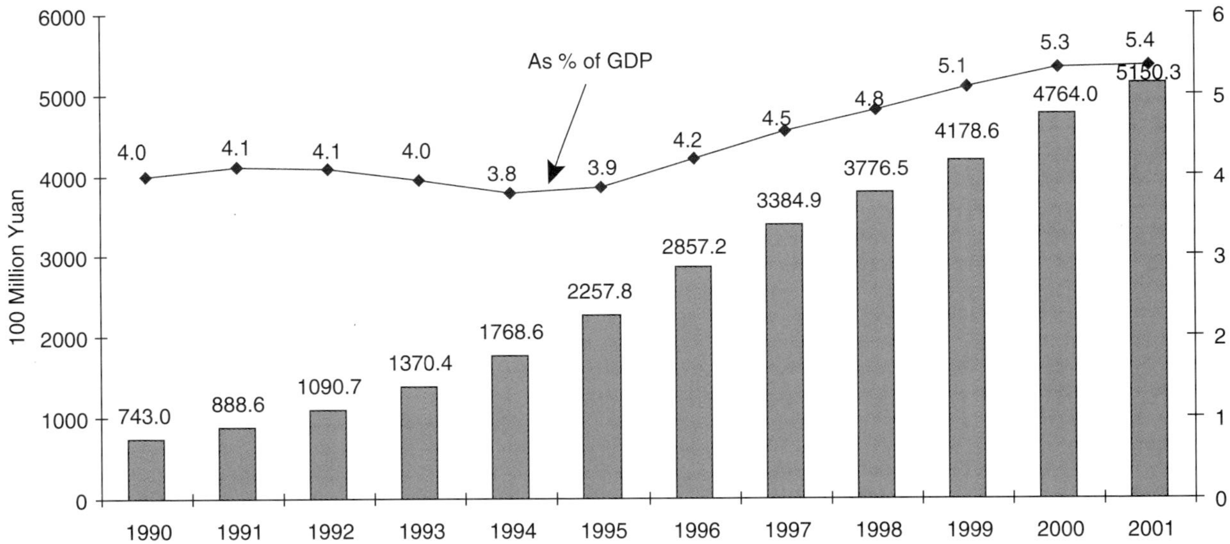

Figure 1. Total Expenditure in China 1990–2001

Sources: *China Health Yearbook*, 2002, p. 503; *China Health Yearbook*, 2001, p. 501; *China Health Statistical Yearbook*, 2003; Zhao, Kun, Guangyin Gao and Quan Wan. 2002. "Report of estimating China's total health expenditures in 2000", *Chinese Health Economics*, Vol. 21, No. 2, pp. 29–32; Li, Yaqing. 2001. "China's total health expenditures: An analysis of their financing sources", *Chinese Health Economics*, Vol. 21, No. 2. pp. 29–30.

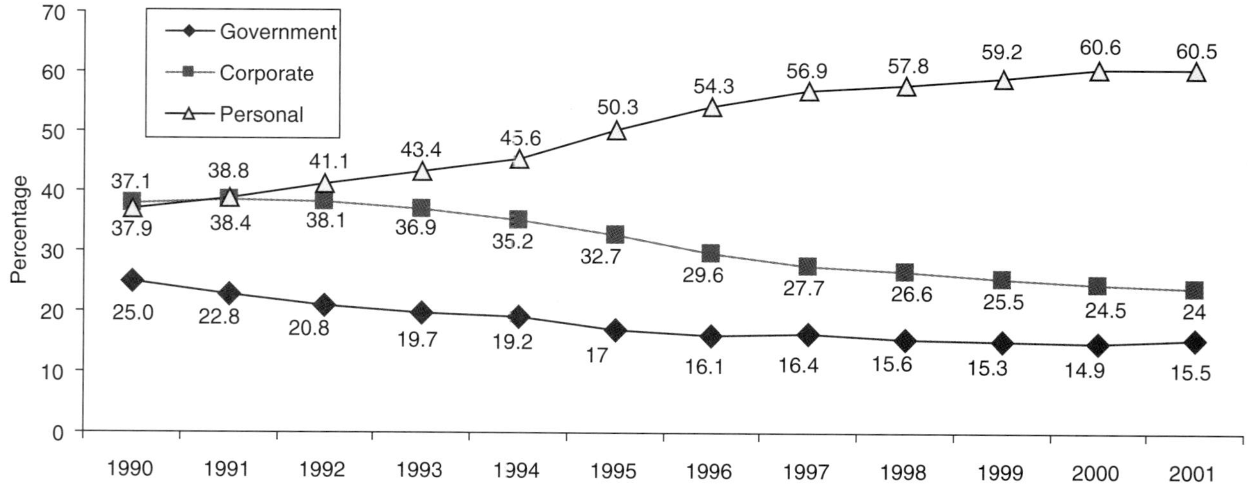

Figure 2. Composition of Total Health Expenditures in China, 1990–2001

Sources: *China Health Yearbook*, 2002, p. 503; *China Health Yearbook*, 2001, p. 501; *China Health Statistical Yearbook*, 2003; Zhao, Kun, Guangyin Gao and Quan Wan. 2002. "Report of estimating China's total health expenditures in 2000", *Chinese Health Economics*, Vol. 21, No. 2, pp. 29–32; Li, Yaqing. 2001. "China's total health expenditures: An analysis of their financing sources", *Chinese Health Economics*, Vol. 21, No. 2. pp. 29–30; *China Statistical Yearbook*, 2003, pp. 53, 320.

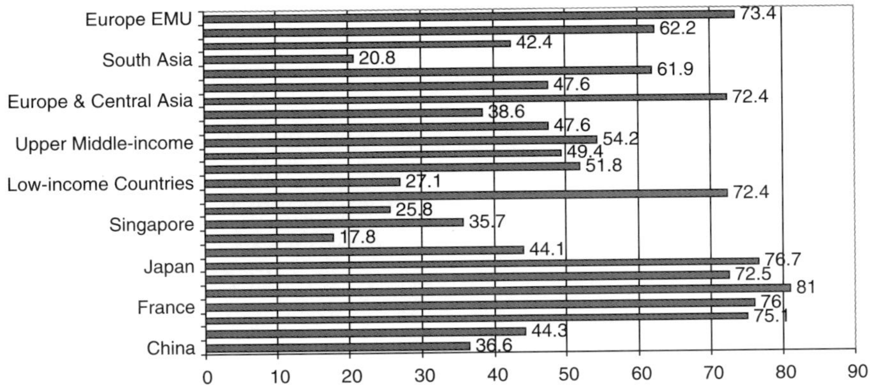

Figure 3. Government Health Expenditure as Percentage of Total Health Expenditure in Selected Countries and Areas, 1997–2000

Source: World Bank. 2003. *2003 World Development Indicators*. Washington, D.C.: The World Bank, pp. 92–94

The objective of this paper is to examine these three aspects in details, as well as to briefly discuss how the Chinese government learnt from this crisis and took steps in improving the health care system. Before doing that, certain reservations need to be made. First, this paper has no intention to produce a comprehensive evaluation of China's crisis management system. To examine this important issue, we need another paper, and scrutinize it under the field of public management. Second, this paper does not discuss general public health challenges brought about by SARS, in particular those common to all countries and regions, as well as medical measures commonly used to deal with the crisis. The detailed discussions of these can be easily found in a variety of professional journals in the fields of epidemiology, public health, and health policy. The target of this paper is the challenges unique to China's healthcare regime. Third, this paper does not go beyond the health sector to touch on the other factors in other fields, in particular those political and economic factors. Discussions on other aspects of the SARS crisis can be found in other chapters of this volume. The purpose of this paper is only to identify certain loopholes in China's healthcare regime, which is vulnerable to public health crisis such as the SARS epidemic.

MEDICAL INSURANCE INEQUALITY AND PUBLIC HEALTH INSECURITY

One of the most significant factors characteristic of the current Chinese healthcare regime is the lack of universal medical insurance coverage. Many uninsured SARS patients were very reluctant to pursue treatment until they were in severe sickness. As a result, they had already become infectors, super- or not, when they had to receive the treatment. The failure of receiving early treatment was one of most important factors for the spread of the SARS virus among the crowd.

Before the economic reforms in late 1978, most Chinese people were covered by medical insurance. In urban areas, the vast majority of working people, retirees, and all university and college students enjoyed free healthcare services. Their family members were also partially protected.[2] In rural areas, Chinese peasants were protected by cooperative medical schemes, jointly financed by the community and the state.[3]

Since the market transition in 1978, however, the insurance coverage rate witnessed a sharp decline. In urban China, healthcare services are no longer free for most of working people since the mid-1990s. Although civil servants still enjoy the free healthcare system, a new social medical insurance system targeting formal employees in enterprises and other kinds of organizations is taking shape. The establishment of this new system has been proceeding very slowly, and so far its coverage is still confined to state-owned enterprises.[4] Commercial health insurance

[2] For more details, among others, see V. W. Sidel and R. Sidel. 1973. *Serving the People: Observations on Medicine in the People's Republic of China*. Boston: Beacon Press; W. Whyte and W. Paris. 1984. *Urban Life in Contemporary China*. Chicago: University of Chicago Press, pp. 62–65; World Bank. 1984. *China: The Health Sector*. Washington, DC.: The World Bank.

[3] For more details, among others, see S. Tang, G. Bloom, X. Feng, H. Lucas, X. Gu, and M. Segall. 1994. *Financing Rural Health Services in China: Adapting to Economic Reform*. IDS Research Report, No. 26, Brighton, UK.: Institute for Developmental Studies; World Bank. 1997. *Financing Health Care: Issues and Options for China*. Washington, DC.: The World Bank.

[4] For more detailed studies of urban health insurance reforms, see Edward Gu. 2001 "Market transition and the transformation of the health care system in urban China", *Policy Studies*, Vol. 22, Nos 3/4, pp. 197–215; and Liu Yuanli. 2002. "Reforming China's urban health insurance system", *Health Policy*, Vol. 60, pp. 133–150.

is also emerging, targeting working people who are not covered by the social insurance system, mainly employees in foreign-invested companies. In rural China, most cooperative medical schemes collapsed during the market transition in the late 1970s.[5] The restoration of the cooperative medical system was set as a policy goal in mid-1990s under the Zhu Rongji administration, but in reality the progress in this regard has been terribly slow due to the government's financial constraint and the deep distrust of peasants towords the government.[6]

As Figure 4 indicates, by 2001, urban residents covered by free healthcare system and health insurance schemes (social or private) accounted

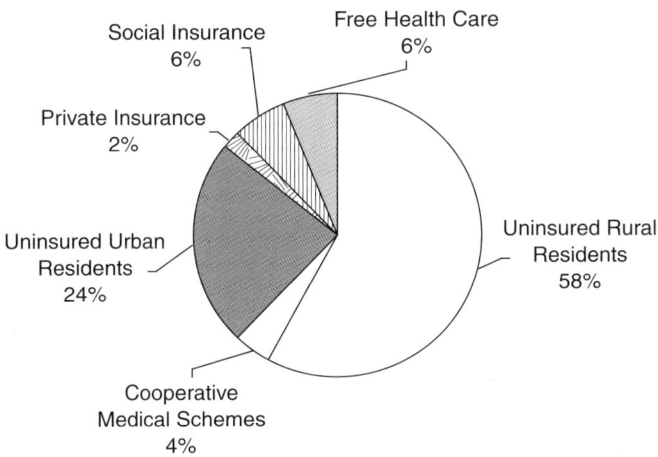

Figure 4. Health Insurance Coverage in China, 2001

Sources: My own estimate, calculated from data of Chinese population and employment in different sectors in terms of ownership. Data are drawn from *Chinese Statistical Yearbook*, 2002.

[5] See Gu Xingyuan, Gerald Bloom, Tang Shenglan, Zhu Yingya, Zhou Shouqi, and Chen Xingbao. 1993. "Financing healthcare in rural China: Preliminary report of a nationwide study", *Social Science and Medicine*, Vol. 36, pp. 385–391.

[6] See Gerald Bloom and Tang Shenglan. 1999. "Rural health prepayment schemes in China: Towards a more active role for government", *Social Science and Medicine*, Vol. 48, pp. 951–960; and Zhang Wenbin. 2003. "Zhongguo nongcun weisheng yiliao baozhang zhidu jianshe lujing" (Approaches to build up health insurance system in rural China), *Chinese Rural Economy*, No. 3, pp. 40–47.

for only 14% of the total population. Only 7% of rural population, or 4% of the total population, were covered by the cooperative medical schemes. The vast majority of Chinese people, namely 82% of the total population, were not protected by any medical insurance schemes. Although 2002–2003 figures are not available yet, the basic structure of medical insurance coverage remains largely unchanged.

The uninsured consists of mainly the peasants and the urban poor. In urban China, a minimum requirement for being covered by social health insurance is urban residence. Many Chinese peasants who are looking for jobs in the cities are not granted the formal (permanent) urban residence, and they are called "peasant workers," "migrant worker", or simply "floating people". A large proportion of these people are employed in the construction sector, and they work and live in terribly crowded conditions.[7] They enjoy no benefits whatsoever.

The uninsured normally does not seek medical treatment promptly when they are getting ill, in particular when they feel that their illness is not severe.[8] One of the important factors contributing to the SARS epidemic is that during its early stage, its symptoms were widely misperceived as flu and therefore patients did not take them seriously. There were indications that the uninsured was reluctant to seek early treatment when they had SARS-like symptoms until the situation worsened. An incomplete statistical analysis of the occupational distribution of SARS patients in China from April 24 to May 25 (see Figure 5) shows that possible uninsured people (comprising "peasant worker", peasants, and, likely, unemployed urban residents) accounted about one-fourth of SARS cases. A further analysis indicates that the proportion of SARS patients who were peasant workers went up towards the end of the epidemic (see Figure 6). Based on interviews with some public health researchers in

[7] Actually, these issues had attracted the attention of the government during the SARS crisis. The Beijing municipal government required all employers who hired a large number of "peasant workers" to improve their working and living conditions, see http://www.chinanews.com.cn/n/2003-04-26/26/298010.html.

[8] Based upon a national survey of health services conducted in 1998, some Chinese health policy researchers found that there was positive correlation between the utilization of healthcare services and health insurance status (see http://www.moh.gov.cn/statistics/ronhs98/index.htm).

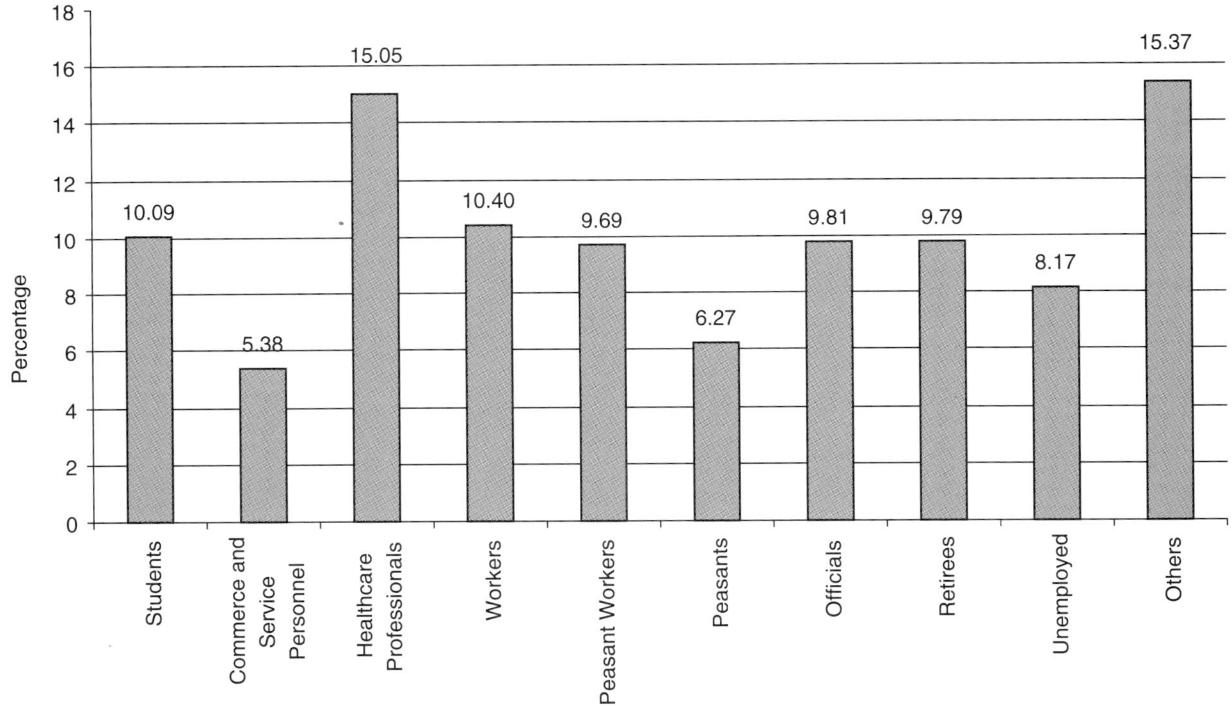

Figure 5. Occupational Distribution of SARS Patients in China, April 24 to May 25

Source: Official websites of China's Ministry of Health, http://www.moh.gov.cn.

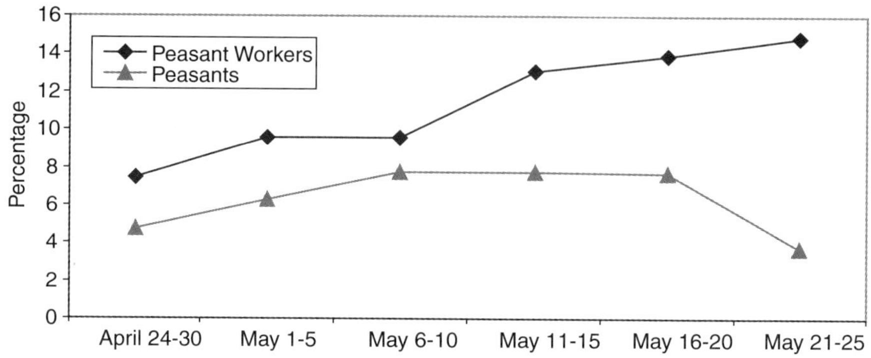

Figure 6. Porportion of SARS Patients Who were Peasant Workers and Peasants Over Different Epidemic Periods

Source: Official website of China's Ministry of Health, http://www.moh.gov.cn.

Beijing after the crisis, my preliminary judgment is that the SARS infection among peasant workers can be largely explained by their poor working and living conditions, but the sharp increase in the number of cases towards the end of the epidemic can be explained only by their behavioral reluctance of receiving early treatment due to financial constraint.

During the SARS epidemic, many officials and scholars, domestic or international, were strongly concerned with the possibility of the SARS spreading to the Chinese countryside.[9] Eventually, the worst situation did not happen, and actually the number of peasants hit by SARS decreased towards the end of the epidemic, largely because peasants live very dispersedly and other rural communities carried out tough social control to prevent any potential SARS virus carriers from entering the villages.[10]

[9] Liu Jian, vice-minister of the Ministry of Agriculture, acknowledged at an official news conference held on May 15, 2003 that it was hard to prevent SARS from spreading to China's rural areas due to the poor conditions of public health system (see http://www.zaobao.com/special/pneumonia/pages1/pneumonia160503s.html).

[10] There were many news reports on how rural communities imposed tough control over the entry of non-community members, especially those coming back from the cities, into their village. Some measures were so tough that they became ridiculous. For instance, a local official in Hebei province ordered the destruction of the road to block any SARS suspects going to his area of jurisdiction. Many peasants in Beijing suburbs set up blockades on road to stop all automobiles from Beijing from going into the suburbs.

The Commercialization of Healthcare Providers and the SARS Crisis

The increasing decline of the state's role in financing the health sector has resulted in the rapid commercialization of healthcare providers at almost all levels, leading to the surge in healthcare costs. As out-of-pocket finance is dominant, soaring costs would definitely drag down the utilization rate of healthcare services. The problem with SARS was that if SARS patients were reluctant or unable to receive treatment in hospitals, they would become infectors.

Before the economic reforms, most Chinese healthcare providers were organized in the public sector. In urban areas, there were Class I, II, III hospitals. Class I hospitals were actually clinics within SOEs and some other large public-sector organizations. In rural areas, the three-tiered structure comprised hospitals at country and township levels, and so-called "healthcare stations" at village level. Except for healthcare stations at the village level in the countryside, all hospitals were financed by the state and their staff were salaried state employees. Healthcare stations were owned and run by the collectivities, namely the People's Communes, and their staffs were mainly so-called "barefoot doctors" who were employed on a part-time basis.[11]

The market transition has driven most Chinese healthcare providers to be increasingly reliant on the service-for-fee mode of operation. Most healthcare providers, including some public health agencies, have been transformed as fee-for-service organizations, although many are still regarded as public-sector organizations. Some still receive subsidies from the state, but overall its portion to the revenue is on the decline. The 2002 statistics show that for government hospitals, government funding accounted for only 10.2% of their total revenues (see Figure 7), down from 15% in 2001. At the same time, privatization of the health sector is under way. Private healthcare organizations have emerged, but on a smaller scale. Most of them are clinics. In urban areas, the former workplace-affiliated clinics have been gradually transformed into community-based

[11] For more details, see World Bank. 1984. *China: The Health Sector*. Washington, D.C.: The World Bank, pp. 33–76; and Marilynn M. Rosenthal. 1987. *Health Care in the People's Republic of China*. Boulder and London: Westview Press, pp. 5–34.

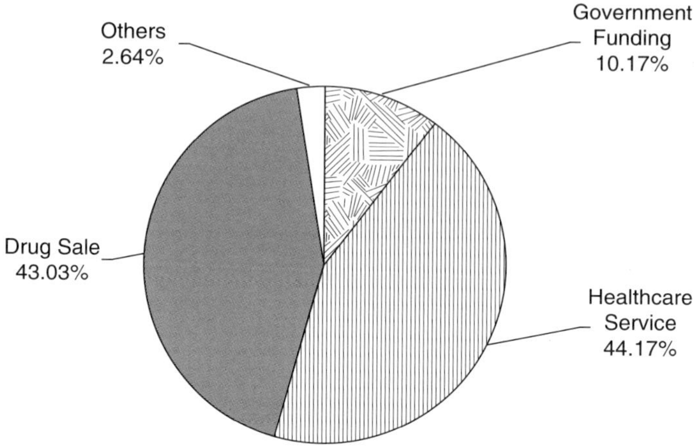

Figure 7. Composition of Government Hospital Revenue, 2002
Source: China Health Statistical Yearbook, 2003.

organizations. In the countryside, there are similar organizations in the village. Recently, plans for privatizing existing public-sector healthcare organizations have been drawn up in the policy agenda.[12]

Under the circumstance, the increase in healthcare costs driven by provider-induced over-consumption is inevitable. As Figure 8 shows, health expenditure per capita grew sharply in the 1990s, and particularly in the late 1990s the growth was accelerated. From 1996 onwards, the growth of health expenditure outpaced the growth of GDP and income. As far as the costs for healthcare services (but rather than more general health expenditure) are concerned, the situation is more severe. Chinese patients now have to have much more money for seeking outpatient and hospitalization services (see Figure 9).

Consequently, the utilization rates of healthcare services are on a decline. The updated data on utilization rates are not available, as the scheduled 2003 national health services survey was delayed due to the SARS crisis. From data collected in the previous national surveys conducted in 1993 and 1998 (see Figure 10), some observations can be made. The utilization of outpatient services in urban areas has increased

[12] Some hospital privatization drives are initiated by local governments.

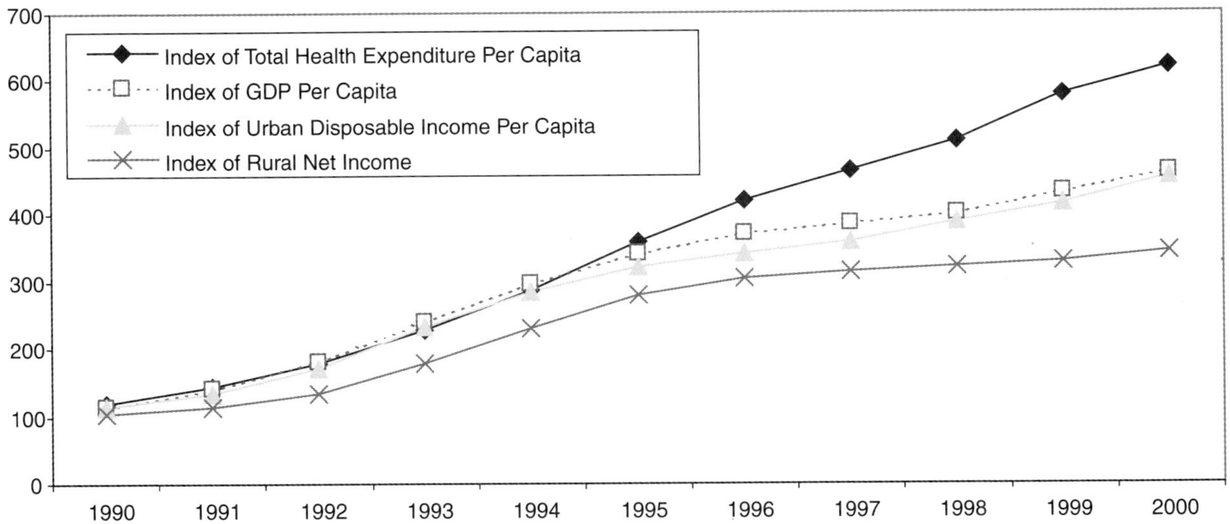

Figure 8. Healthcare Cost Growth in China, Compared with Income Growth, 1995–2001

Sources: China Health Yearbook, 2002, p. 503; *China Health Yearbook*, 2001, p. 501; *China Health Statistical Yearbook*, 2003; Zhao Kun, Gao Guangyin and Wan Quan. 2002. "Report of estimating China's total health expenditures in 2000", *Chinese Health Economics*, Vol. 21, No. 2, pp. 29–32; Li Yaqing. 2001. "China's total health expenditures: An analysis of their financing sources", *Chinese Health Economics*, Vol. 21, No. 2, pp. 29–30; *China Statistical Yearbook*, 2003, pp. 53, 320.

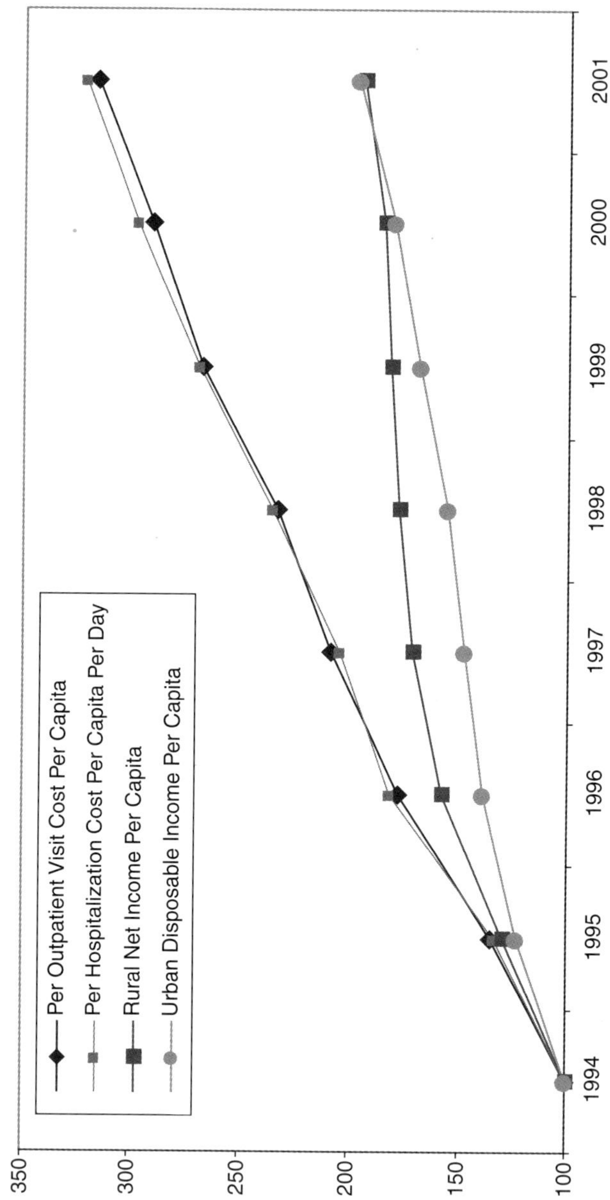

Figure 9. Index Growth of Healthcare Service Costs, Compared with Income Growth, 1994–2001

Sources: China Health Statistical Yearbook, various years; *China Statistical Yearbook*, 2002, p. 320.

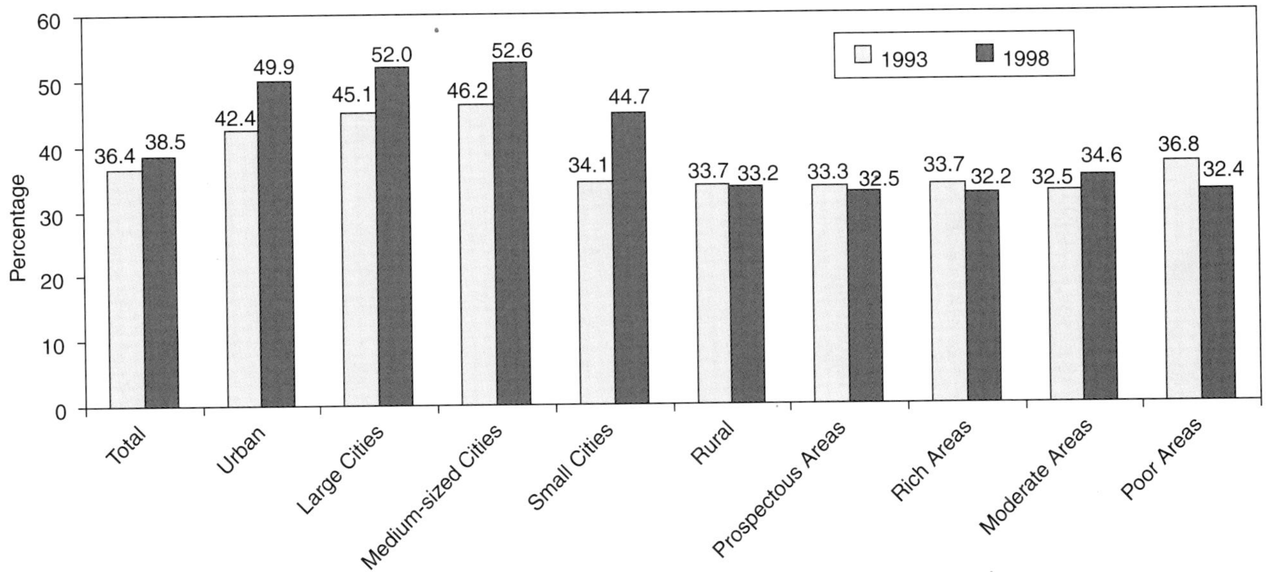

Figure 10. Percentage of Chinese Patients Who Did Not Seek Outpatient Services in 1993 and 1998

Sources: Chinese National Health Service Survey, 1993; 1998. Reports of these two surveys (Chinese versions) can be found at http://www.moh.gov.cn/tjxxzx.ztyjjbg/index.htm.

considerably, in particular with sharper growth in small cities. In rural areas, by contrast, it was a totally different story. Except for moderately rich areas, the utilization rates of outpatient services went down. Similar trends can be also discerned for the utilization of hospitalization services (see Figure 11). For concrete reasons for not seeking healthcare services, the percentage of respondent who clicked financial constraint increased in 1998 in comparison with the situation of 1993 (see Figures 12 and 13). Here, it is worth noting that health insurance reforms were yet to be launched in urban areas during the time of the 1998 survey, when many urban residents still enjoyed free healthcare services. Therefore, it is not difficult to understand that the utilization rates of healthcare services in urban areas did not decrease at that time. Since healthcare services are no longer free from 1998 onwards, the situation would change. It is widely anticipated that the utilization rates of both outpatient and hospitalization services would decrease in both rural and urban areas in recent years.

The impact of the increasing commercialization of healthcare providers on the SARS epidemic is threefold. First, as health services become increasingly unaffordable to many Chinese people, many SARS cases failed to get early treatment. It is unknown as to what extent the reluctance of seeking healthcare services due to financial constraint could constitute a direct contributing factor to the SARS epidemic, as currently available studies of SARS cases are normally confined to the field of epidemiology, rather than in the field of public health policy. But some news reports released during the SARS epidemic unveiled that many patients with fever did not receive adequate medical attention as they could not afford the costly lung examination.[13] In fact, to combat this problem, some municipal governments announced that all confirmed SARS

[13] One of the high-profile stories was that a patient with SARS syndromes escaped from the Anzhen Hospital in Beijing when he was asked to make payment. The authorities found him within one hour through social mobilization. This patient enjoyed free treatment, and eventually he was diagnosed as a case of pulmonary tuberculosis. A spokesman of the Beijing municipal government reiterated when commenting this story that all low-income SARS or SARS-like patients were eligible for applying free treatment. He emphasized that nobody would be declined for treatment due to the failure of making payment (see http://news.nen.com.cn/72340168526266368/20030601/1155370.shtml).

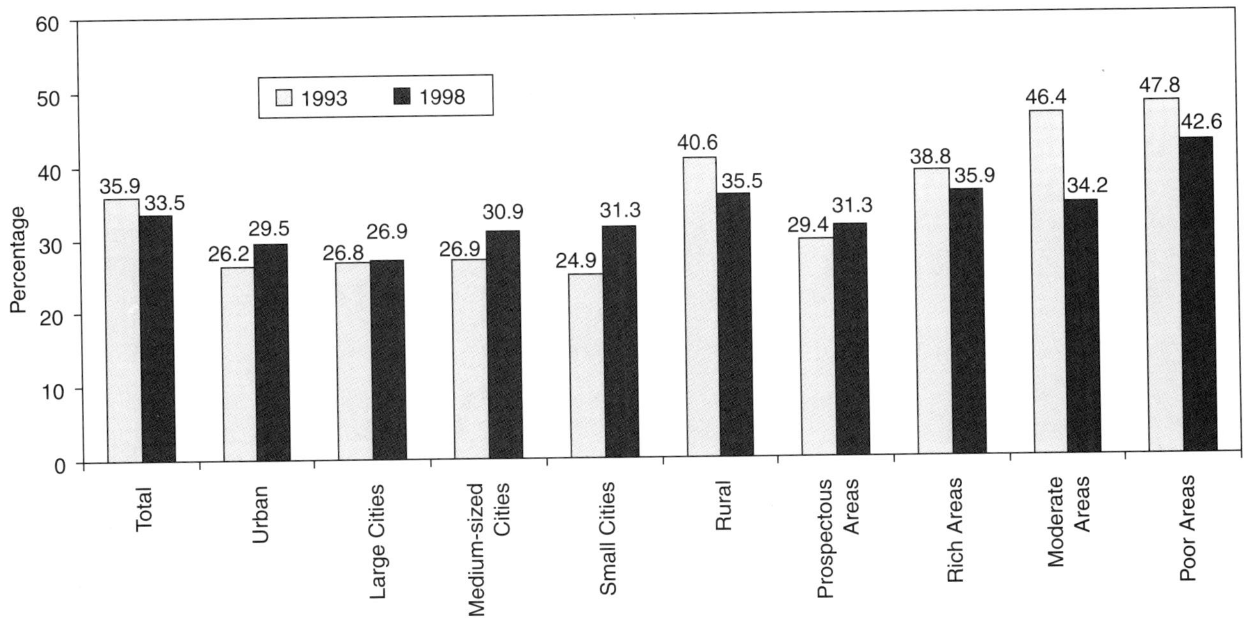

Figure 11. Non-Hospitalization Rates in 1993 and 1998 by Areas

Sources: *Chinese Health Statistical Yearbook*, 1999; *Chinese National Health Survey*, 1993; 1998. The reports of these two surveys (Chinese versions) can be found at http://www.moh.gov.cn/tjxxzx/ztyjjbg/index.htm.

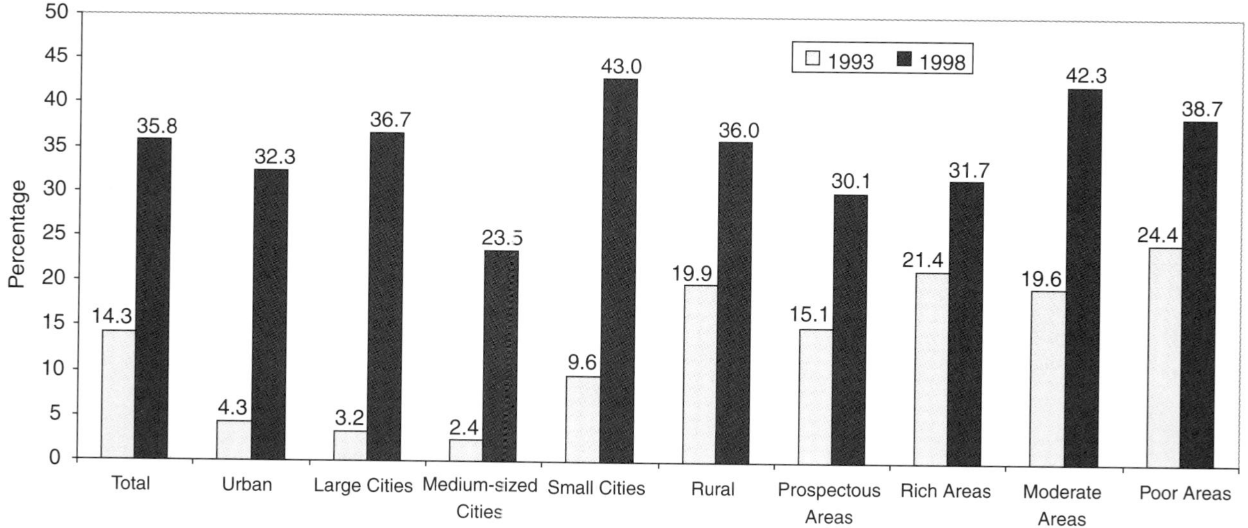

Figure 12. Percentage of Chinese People Who Did Not Seek Outpatient Services Due to Financial Constraint in 1993 and 1998

Sources: *Chinese National Health Service Survey*, 1993; 1998. Reports of these two surveys (Chinese versions) can be found at http://www.moh.gov.cn/tjxxzx/ztyjjbg/index.htm.

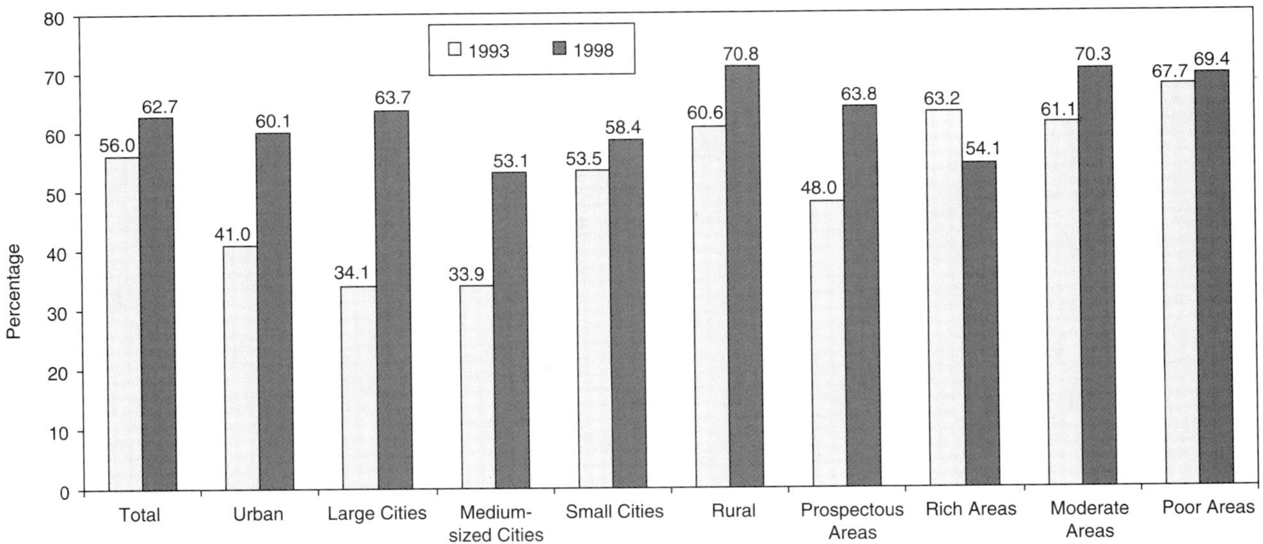

Figure 13. Percentage of Chinese Patients Who Did Not Want to Be Hospitalized Due to Financial Constraint in 1993 and 1998

Sources: Chinese National Health Service Survey, 1993; 1998. The reports of these two surveys (Chinese versions) can be found at http://www.moh.gov.cn/tjxxzx/ztyjjbg/index.htm.

patients would receive free treatment.[14] Wen Jiabao, Premier of China, also announced on May 6, 2003 that all expenses for SARS treatment would be waived for peasants.[15] When he paid an inspection visit to Sichuan's rural areas, Wen Jiabao urged local officials to notify every peasant of the free treatment for SARS. He even advertised this policy on the TV by emphasizing that all expenses including meals and accommodation would be free.

Second, the commercialization of healthcare providers has induced hospitals to restructure their operations towards high revenue-generating services. As a matter of fact, infectious diseases were kept well under control before the outbreak of the SARS crisis. From 1985 to 2002, the reported incidence and death rate of infectious diseases were both kept at low levels (see Figure 14). As a result, the utilization rates of hospital beds in infectious disease and tuberculosis hospitals decreased more drastically than that of the general trend (see Figure 15). In response to this situation, few Chinese hospitals invested in infectious as well as tuberculosis departments over the past years before the SARS epidemic. Figure 16 shows that the number of hospital beds in infectious and tuberculosis departments declined remarkably from 1978 to 2002. Apart from this, the existing infectious and tuberculosis departments tended to be poorly facilitated. According to some news reports, there were no efficient respirators in many hospitals, and nurses were also not well trained to use these machines.[16]

[14] Among them were Wuhan, Chengdu, Fuzhou, and so on. Actually, the number of SARS cases in these cities was not so high that the local government would feel it affordable to deliver free treatment for SARS patients. But in Shanxi where the number of SARS cases was large, the local government promised that only patients who were in poor financial conditions could be eligible for free treatment, and all the expenses would be covered by the government (see http://www.chinanews.com.cn/n/2003-04-26/26/297988.html).

[15] See http://big5.xinhuanet.com/gate/big5/news.xinhuanet.com/misc/2003-05/06/content_859886.htm.

[16] This happened in many general hospitals in Taiyuan, Shanxi Province, which was hit severely by SARS. See "SARS Diaocha: Yichang kongqian zhainan de quanjing shilu" (Investigating SARS: A panorama of an unprecedented catastrophe), *Finance*, pp. 37–79.

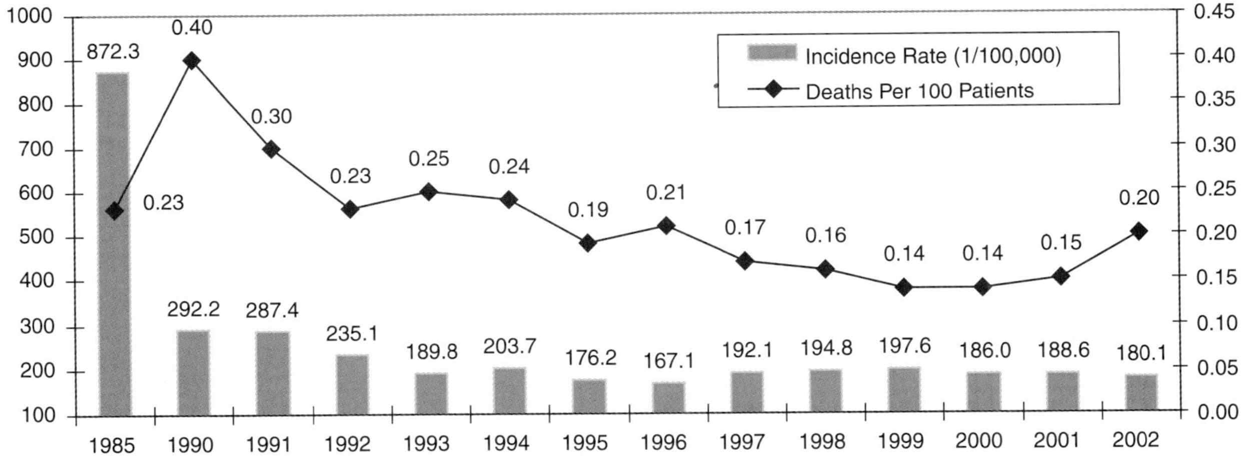

Figure 14. Reported Incidence and Death Rate of Infectious Diseases, 1985–2002

Sources: *China Health Statistical Yearbook*, various years.

Note: Nineteen diseases were reported before 1990. During the period from 1990 to 1995, twenty-four diseases were reported. From 1995 to 2002, two diseases were added to the list of reporting requirement. In May 2003, SARS was added during its outbreak.

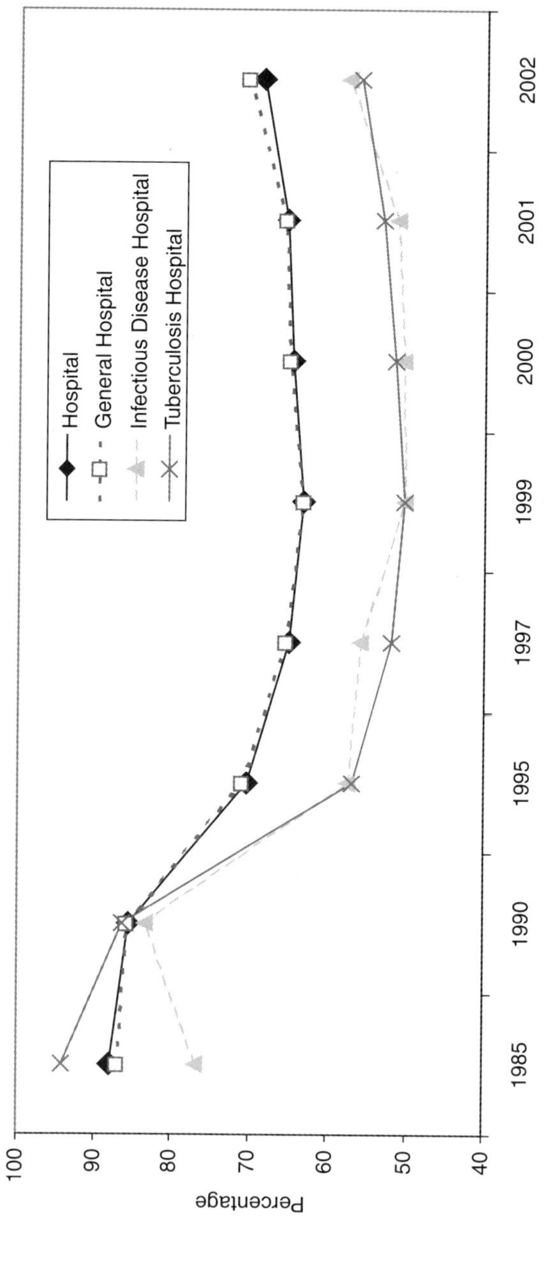

Figure 15. Utilization Rates of Hospital Beds, 1985–2002

Sources: China Health Statistical Yearbook, various years.

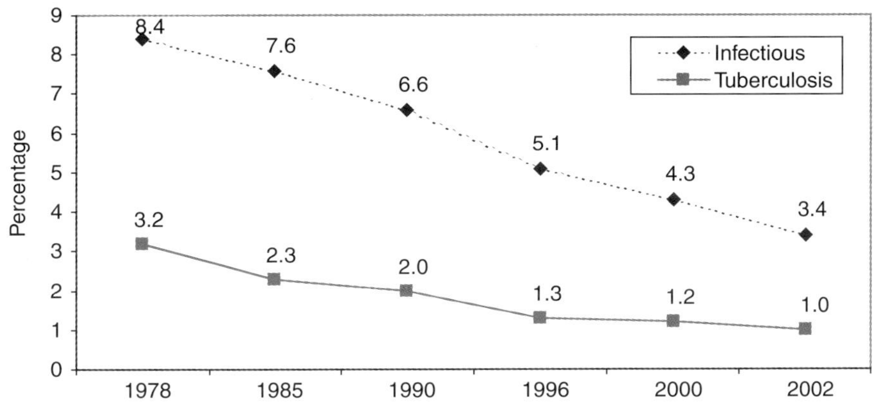

Figure 16. Porportion of Hospital Beds in Infectious and Tuberculosis Departments, Selected Years, 1978–2002

Sources: *China Health Statistical Yearbook*, various years.

Third, as hospitals heavily rely on the revenue generated from their provision of healthcare services, there was a strong incentive for their concealment of the SARS cases and their refusal of treating uninsured SARS suspects. These were particularly manifested during the early period of the SARS epidemic.[17] At that time, local officials were also inclined to conceal the truth of the SARS epidemic out of their concern with potential sabotage of local image as attractive sites for investment and business.[18]

An Ailing Public Health System Exposed in the SARS Crisis

The most direct link between the increasing declining role of the state in financing the health sector and the outbreak of SARS is an ailing public health system. As a result of underinvestment from the state, many public

[17] According to some overseas reports, some hospitals in Beijing attempted to conceal the number of SARS cases during the visit of the WHO inspection team. It is widely believed that the soaring number of SARS cases in Beijing after the sacking of Zhang Wenkang, then Minister of Health, and Meng Xuenong, then Mayor of Beijing, on April 20 was an indication of widespread concealment, although the Chinese authorities denied this.

[18] The concealment was especially evident in Guangdong during the early stages of the crisis. For more details on this, see Lai Hongyi's chapter in this volume.

health agencies are inclined to concentrate on carrying out service-for-fee activities, rather than providing preventive healthcare services.

China has a huge public health system, which consists of various organizations at different levels. Although many hospitals concentrate on providing curative healthcare services, curative and preventive healthcare services are integrated at grassroots levels in urban community hospitals and rural health stations.[19] The most important public health organizations operating in the field of preventive healthcare services are Centers for Disease Control and Prevention, which are formerly called "anti-epidemic stations" and recently renamed as CDCs following the U.S. model. Apart from these centers, there are some specialized agents in charge of public health programs targeting at certain specific infectious diseases.

For a long time, the governance of Chinese CDCs was decentralized. All CDCs were administered by local health bureaux had no efficient mechanism to coordinate and disseminate information across localities. In response to this, the Chinese government re-centralize the system by restructuring the Academy of Preventive Medicine into a new public health agency at the national level, namely Chinese Center for Disease Control and Prevention, in January 2002.[20] The Center undertakes the duties as follows:

- Policy consultation on public health laws, regulations, and policies;
- Planning, implementing, and evaluating public health projects, in particular targeting disease control and prevention;
- Establishment of a national public health surveillance system to monitor environmental hygiene at the workplace;
- Establishment of a public health emergency response system to tackle any emergent public health crisis;
- Vaccine research and production, and the implementation of vaccination projects;

[19] Liu Xingzhu and Anne Mills. 2002. "Financing reforms of public health services in China: Lessons for other nations," *Social Science and Medicine*, Vol. 54, pp. 1691–1698.
[20] See The Chronology of the Chinese Center for Disease Control and Prevention, at http://www.chinacdc.net.cn/view_news/home.cbs?db=zxdsj.

- Reconstruction of drinking water supply in rural areas;
- Scientific research related to public health;
- Training of public health professionals; and
- International public health cooperation.

Despite the huge number of public health organizations and the heavy duties they bear, government spending on public health has been in sharp decline over the past years. Previously, almost all public health agencies were completely financed by the government, and many public health services including preventive services and public health inspections were provided to users free of charge. When economic reforms were launched, these public health agencies joined a wide range of other organizations to transform themselves into service-for-fee organizations. Trends in the sources of their finance are characterized by a decreasing share from the government and an increasing share from service charges.[21] Official statistical data show that from 1995 onwards government spending on public health, measured by its percentage of total health expenditure and its proportion in the government health expenditure, decreased sharply (see Figure 17), although the latter indicator has recently seen a slight rebound from its lowest level in 1997. As a result of the declining government spending on the public health sector, the number of salaried physicians in CDCs recorded a slower growth than the total number of physicians in the health sector (see Figure 18).

The financing reforms of China's public health system have produced a twofold consequence. On the one hand, the introduction of an economic incentive that links service provision with revenue has provided a strong stimulus to the productivity and efficiency of the sector. On the other hand, most public health agencies have shifted their focus on revenue-generating public health services, resulting in the underprovision of services with public goods' characteristics.[22] Among revenue-generating services are health screening and public health inspections, while disease control, vaccination and public health education are among the services that are unlikely to

[21] Liu and Mills. "Financing reforms of public health services in China", pp. 1691–1698.
[22] *Ibid.*, pp. 1694–1695.

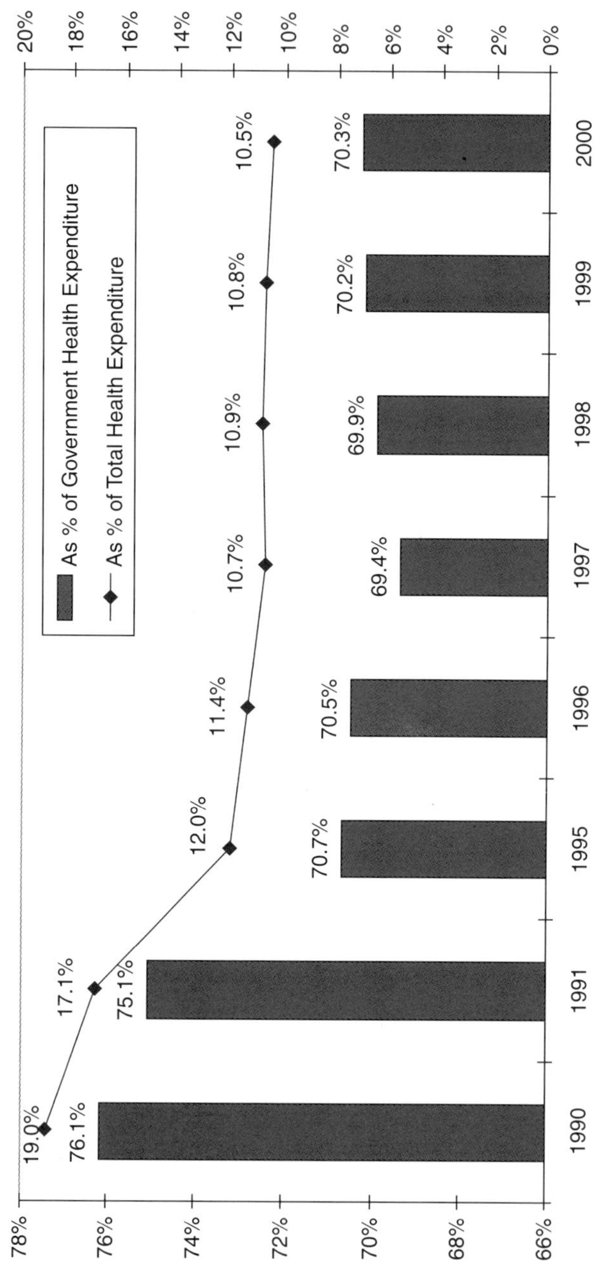

Figure 17. Government Spending on Public Health in China, 1990–2000

Sources: China Health Statistical Yearbook, various years.

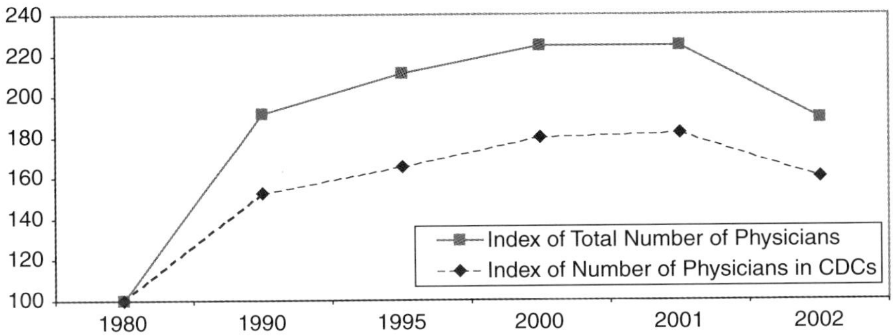

Figure 18. Growth in Number of Physicians in CDCs Compared with Growth in Total Number, 1980–2002

Sources: *China Health Statistical Yearbook*, various years.

generate much revenue.[23] In contextualizing the SARS crisis within the background of public health financing reforms, it would not be difficult to understand how such a public health system deemphasizing disease control could be terribly hit by the outbreak of a new disease.

A more direct link between an ailing China's public health system and the SARS crisis lies with the poor mechanism of information dissemination. A well-functioning information dissemination subsystem is obviously critical to crisis management. Such a system was obviously not in place when SARS hit the country, although its establishment was set as a goal for the Chinese Center for Disease Control and Prevention. There are two reasons for this sluggishness: on the one hand, the Center had been established less than a year when SARS occurred in Guangdong; on the other its capacity building proceeded slowly largely because the government had failed to provide efficient funding.

The consequence of this sluggishness was disastrous indeed. The poor coordination within the public health system and the disintegration between public and personal health care sectors were some of the major reasons for the SARS outbreak. Actually, public health professionals in

[23] Liu Guoxiang, Zhao Yuqin, Li Yaqing and Du Lexun. 2001. "Zhongguo weisheng fangyizhan feiyong cesuan fangfa yu cesuan jieguo yanjiu" (Measuring public health expenditures by CDCs in China and examining the results), *Chinese Health Economics*, Vol. 20, No. 5, pp. 37–39.

Guangdong had already reported the SARS cases to the Chinese Center for Disease Control and Prevention and the Ministry of Health as early as February 2003, but it seemed that no guidelines or precautious measures were established until April 20 when Zhang Wenkang, the then Minister of Health, was sacked. In Beijing, Taiyuan, and other cities, many doctors had to mobilize their personal connections to collect relevant information on SARS from their colleagues in Guangdong.[24]

The problem of poor coordination and information dissemination within the health sector was further enhanced due to the separation of the military and the civilian healthcare provision. It was widely believed that during the early stage of the SARS epidemic, one of the major reasons for the Beijing municipal government's ignorance of accurate number of SARS cases was that the army's hospitals did not report their cases to the local authorities.[25]

Temporary Measures and Long-term Commitments: Towards a More Active Role for the State

As the ailing healthcare system could not handle the SARS crisis, the Chinese government eventually stepped in to restore many measures prevalent in the old regime. The virtue of social mobilization and control with authoritarian and even totalitarian characteristics were rediscovered. In brief, the government's intervention fell into the categories as follows:[26]

- Enhancing government leadership and speeding up legislature: (1) national headquarters to combat the crisis established (for its structure, see Figure 19); (2) inspections teams sent to all provinces

[24] According to some reports, many doctors in Beijing and Taiyuan knew little about SARS or the possibly feasible treatments used in Guangdong when the first batch of SARS patients was received. As a result, the number of SARS cases in hospitals and especially among healthcare professionals soared. See "Investigating SARS", pp. 110–113.

[25] This phenomenon of institutional fragmentation was openly criticized by some WHO officials at a news conference held on April 16, 2003. See "Investigating SARS", p. 35.

[26] The following is summarized from a speech delivered by Gao Qiang, Deputy Minister of Health to the International Conference on SARS Control and Prevention held on June 17, 2003 in Kuala Lumpur.

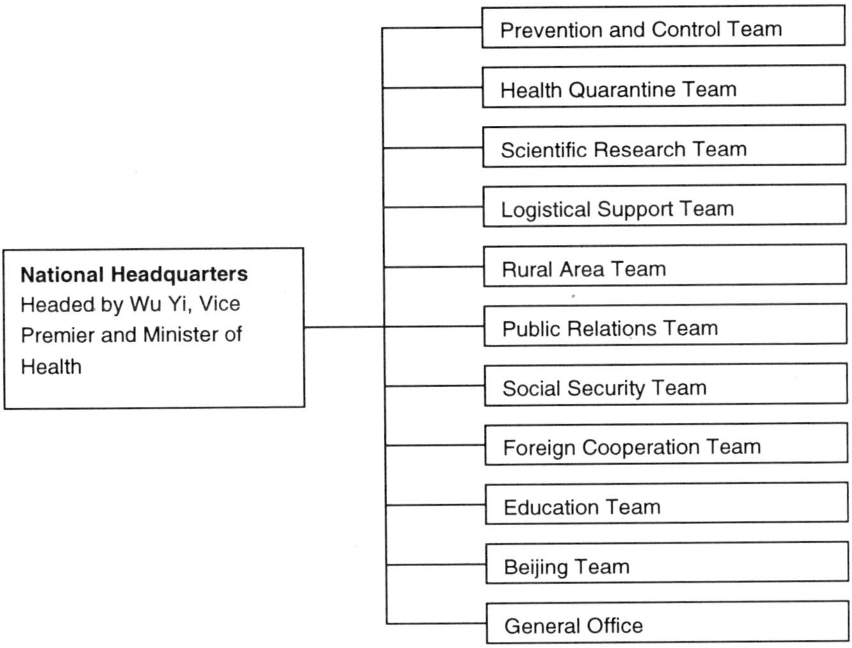

Figure 19. The Structure of China's National Headquarters to Combat the SARS Crisis

by the State Council, and similar teams sent to all levels of the government to monitor the local struggle against SARS; and (3) the existing law on control and prevention of infectious diseases amended, and new regulations on public health emergence alert and response in general and on SARS control and prevention issued.

- Establishing an effective surveillance and information system: (1) a national disease reporting and information management system established since April 20, 2003; and (2) a rural surveillance system set up connecting local officials and healthcare professionals at village, township, and county levels.
- Imposing strict infection control in communities: (1) peasants in villages and towns mobilized to build up mass defence lines; (2) urban neighborhood committees (community-based, semi-governmental organizations) organized to monitor probable SARS cases among residents in general and mobile population (i.e., "peasant workers") in particular; and (3) workplace units in cities mobilized to impose

precautionary measures, propagate civil education on public hygiene, and impose quarantine.

- Restoring certain old-regime measures with healthcare services: (1) a central government special fund set up to provide free SARS treatment, including meals during hospitalization and quarantine, for all peasants and the urban poor; (2) tough administrative control over all healthcare providers resumed; (3) medical infrastructure and expertise in hospitals upgraded through government financing; and (4) a specific hospital for treating SARS patients, namely Xiaotangshan Hospital, built up within one week of mobilizing the support from the military.

All these measures were temporary in nature. They were to some extent effective, given the poor public health infrastructure and the large scale of infected population in China. It is inevitable that some irregularities could occur in such a large country. One of the major fields in which such irregularities are taking place is resource allocation. Many hospitals in SARS-hit cities and some rural hospital providers are complaining loudly that their revenues for normal operation have been exhausted by carrying out SARS treatment and precautionary vaccines. Although a special SARS relief fund had been set up by the central government, the negotiation between different health providers, local governments, and the central government over how to allocate these funds is still under way. Many severely hit hospitals are now relying on bank loans for their operation.[27]

It is widely recognized, explicitly or implicitly, that political campaign and social mobilization cannot be carried out all the time, unless China would be prepared to go back to the totalitarian-revolutionary era.[28] To prevent similar public health crisis from reoccurring, China has to improve its healthcare regime. Actually, the SARS outbreak has prompted the Chinese government to reconsider its role in the health

[27] For reports on poor financial situations with many hospitals in affected areas such as Shanxi, Hebei, and Inner Mongolia, see "Investigating SARS", pp. 37–67.

[28] The best study of social mobilization during China's totalitarian-revolutionary era is Tang Tsou. 1986. *The Cultural Revolution and Post-Mao Reforms: A Historic Perspective*. Chicago: University of Chicago Press.

sector. The call for re-examining, or even abandoning, the marketing approach to health reforms arises during the aftermath of the crisis.[29] The Chinese government has learnt bitter lessons from playing down the importance of investing in social infrastructure, and is planning to take some long-term measures to reconfigure its public health system in particular and the whole healthcare regime in general. The measures would be taken at least in the fields as follows:

- Increasing investment in public health;
- Establishing a public health emergence alert and response system;
- Improving disease control system;
- Strengthening healthcare system, especially in rural areas.

The measures taken in the first three fields have bolstered the government's investment in public health. Although the overall figures on government spending are not available as the fiscal year has not yet passed, it is pretty sure that a large proportion of newly increased government spending on public health has been channelled to SARS-related research and capacity-building within the CDC establishment.[30] A major step taken is the establishment of a national SARS information dissemination system. On October 17, 2003, the Ministry of Health tested this new system across the nation. By the date, about 10,800 hospitals (among 15,000) at the county and the above levels and 8,000 township hospitals (among about 50,000) had been connected through this system. The government's goal for improving this system is to achieve 100% coverage in the cities and considerably upgrade the coverage rate in rural areas by the end of 2003.[31]

[29] For example, Wang Shaguang and Hu Angang, working together with their assistants, published a number of influential papers criticizing the marketizing approach to health reforms in China. Most of their papers are available from Hu Angang, ed. 2003. *Toushi SARS: Jiankang yu Fazhan* (*SARS in Perspectives: Health and Development*). Beijing: Tsinghua Univeristy Press.

[30] Hu Jintao emphasized on April 20, 2003 the importance of scientific research in the battle against SARS (see http://big5.xinhuanet.com/gate/big5/news.xinhuanet.com/newscenter/2003-04/20/content_841011.htm).

[31] The news is available at http://news.sina.com.cn/c/2003-10-17/1301935606s.shtml.

The government in pursuing a more active role in improving China's ailing health regime is indeed a long-term commitment. One of the priorities on the policy agenda is to improve healthcare financing in rural areas.[32] Actually, the Chinese government was shocked when the World Health Organization's 2000 report *Improving Health Systems* ranked China as 196 among 199 members with regard to the fairness of health financing. A major factor leading to this low ranking is the lack of functioning rural healthcare financing system. Within this context, the Chinese government which is very concerned with its international image has decided to push forward the long delayed plan of restoring cooperative medical insurance system in rural areas.[33] Yet progress has been so sluggish that it is still in the stage of small-scaled experiments due to many reasons such as fiscal constraints for the governments at all levels, the tough choice between individual medical savings account or a social insurance system, the design of benefit structure, and the poor knowledge among Chinese peasants of insurance.

The SARS crisis gave the Chinese government another shock. During the crisis it was reiterated by Chinese leaders and some WHO officers that if the SARS epidemic were to spread to the countryside, it would be more disastrous. Actions are being taken on two fronts. One is to expand the experiments with cooperative medical system. On June 16 and 17, 2003, when the war against SARS was yet to claim victory, the Ministry of Health organized a workshop for local officials in charge of the experiments on rural cooperative medical system to share experiences and lessons.[34] On October 14 and 15, 2003, Wu Yi, the Minister of Health, presided over another working conference on the rural cooperative medical system where the decision of expanding and accelerating the experiments was announced.

[32] The description is based on my conversations with many officials and policy researchers during my fieldwork on China's health reforms in September and October.

[33] The WHO report was published in 2000, but the research for this report was conducted in 1997. Many Chinese official policy researchers took part in the research, and therefore the research findings were already available to them by that time.

[34] For the details of this workshop, see http://www.moh.gov.cn/jcwsyfybj/1200308080007.htm .

Another is the establishment of a medical assistance system in both rural and urban areas. As a matter of fact, a variety of medical assistance schemes, similar with the U.S. Medicaid model, has been established in some economically prosperous cities and suburban areas, e.g., Shanghai, Guangzhou, and many cities in Zhejiang province. The Ministry of Civil Affairs is gathering domestic and international experts to investigate these local initiatives in order to design institutional arrangements applicable to all cities. Meanwhile, the central government has committed 300,000,000 RMB from the 2004 budget to set up a rural medical assistance system. Currently, the Ministry of Civil Affairs is mobilizing experts to draft the regulations.[35]

In Chinese, the word "crisis" could deliver two meanings, namely disaster and opportunity. The SARS crisis was indeed calamitous, but it provided an opportunity to China. All societal actors who are concerned with social development and social justice have found a new context to justify their claims and appeal to the public. Likewise, all state actors who are in charge of social affairs, in particular those who are in charge of public health and social welfare policies, have found a new lever to strengthen their bargaining power over resource allocation against their counterparts within the Party-state establishment. More important, the new Chinese leadership, headed by President and Party Chairman Hu Jintao and Premier Wen Jiabao, have found a new platform, symbolically, to build a new image in ruling style, and, substantially, to carry out certain policy shift towards more emphasis on sustainable and balanced socioeconomic development in China.

[35] The author was among invited experts to provide consultation on drafting the regulations.

Chapter 6

"Chinese Scientists were Defeated by SARS"*[1]

CAO CONG

> ... many scientists here are saddened at losing an opportunity to show off China's growing scientific prowess. Chinese scientists could have been the first to nail the pathogen, sequence its genome, and describe how it sickens its victims.
>
> MARTIN ENSERINK[2]

The outbreak of an epidemic involves scientific, medical, and public health issues. From a pure scientific research perspective, it calls for the identification of the cause of the disease, or the detection of pathogen, the finding of the way it transmits, and eventually the development of vaccines; clinically, it needs to diagnose the probable, or confirmed, cases as

* Fieldwork for this paper was supported by a research grant (R348-000-005-112) from the Faculty of Arts and Social Sciences, the National University of Singapore. The revision of the essay has benefited from the comments made by participants at "SARS and Governance in China," a workshop held at the East Asian Institute, the National University of Singapore, and by Professors Jonathan R. Cole and Richard P. Suttmeier.

[1] This is a remark made by Yang Huanming, director of the Beijing Genomics Institute (BGI), then a non-governmental research institute, that would become part of the Chinese Academy of Sciences amid the SARS episode, reportedly to Hu Jintao, the general secretary of the Chinese Communist Party Central Committee and China's state president. See Xie Xiang and Zhou Xinyu. "Yang Huanming's pain" (in Chinese), *China Youth News*, 26 May 2003.

[2] Martin Enserink. "China's missed chance", *Science*, Vol. 301 (18 Jul 2003), pp. 294–296.

early, fast, and accurate as possible, develop standard treatment protocols, reduce mortality rate, and so on; and the prevention of the disease from spreading to communities challenges public health professionals. All these require the collaboration between scientists and medical doctors, the mobilization and best use of resources, and the cooperation of the public.

The crisis of severe acute respiratory syndrome (SARS) between the winter of 2002 and the summer of 2003 in China was a serious test for its scientific, medical, and public health capabilities to handle an emergency. Although to some extent it is the politicization of SARS to blame — China attempted to sweep the SARS epidemic under the rug at the beginning,[3] the Chinese scientific and medical community failed the test, or in the words of Yang Huanming, one of the examinees, "Chinese scientists were defeated by SARS". In retrospect, despite mainland China being the *first* country to witness the disease, having the most cases, and having the lowest death rate among the SARS patients in the world, its scientists have not registered any *first* in the international competition for priority in the fight against the disease. The isolation and identification of the pathogen of SARS — a new variety of coronavirus — went to scientists in Hong Kong; Canadian scientists first sequenced the genomes of the virus; most recently, scientists outside mainland China have started to compare genomic sequences obtained from different SARS viral strains to figure out the differences and mutations, and published their epidemiological research on the SARS outbreak.

The occurrence of SARS in China presents a good opportunity to examine the issues that the Chinese scientific community has been facing in the reform era, such as organizational characteristics, incentives and motivations for scientific research, power and influence of the elite, scientific communications, and so on. The essay is going to examine how China's scientific and medical community responded to the SARS crisis and why they lost the battle through three case studies. In particular, it examines how the authoritative structure prevented Chinese scientists from early detection of the cause of the disease, why scientists from different jurisdictions did not collaborate, and why they failed to

[3] See, for example, Joseph Fewsmith. "China and the politics of SARS", *Current History*, (September 2003), pp. 250–255.

communicate their knowledge gathered in the SARS research and the treatment of SARS patients to the international scientific community. The essay will also point out that the problematic practices during that period have persisted, which might lead to further problems.

Hong Tao, China's National CDC, and the Chlamydia Hypothesis

In November 2002, the first case of a mystery illness occurred in Guangdong province, which caused a severe panic during the Chinese New Year of 2003. On February 11, 2003, the Guangdong Health Bureau held the first press conference on the matter in Guangzhou, the capital city of Guangdong, disclosing that there had been 305 cases of a mystery aliment with five deaths in the province. According to the health officials, the provincial and national centers for disease control and prevention (CDC) had ruled out the possibility that the disease is anthrax, plague, or bird influenza. During that press conference, Dr. Zhong Nanshan, director of the Guangzhou Institute of Respiratory Disease affiliated to the Guangzhou Medical College and a prestigious member (*yuanshi*) of the Chinese Academy of Engineering (CAE) who would later be known to the world for his role in combating SARS, named the disease "atypical pneumonia" which was most likely caused by a virus.[4] Also on that day, the first SARS patient autopsy in China as well as in the world was performed at Nanfang Hospital, a military hospital in Guangzhou, and tissue samples from the autopsy were then distributed among the Guangdong CDC, Guangzhou CDC, and the Guangzhou No. 8 People's Hospital that contributed the corpse.[5] On February 12, Nanfang Hospital attributed the death to a virus-caused pneumonia.

[4] Liao Huailing. "The victory of the honesty: The identification of the SARS pathogen as coronavirus" (in Chinese), http://www.peopledaily.com.cn/GB/shehui/212/10548/10649/20030517/994571.html, accessed on 17 May 2003.

[5] Zhang Jing. "SARS attacked China's research management system" (in Chinese), *Twenty-First Century Economic News*, 12 Jun 2003. The disease was later named SARS following the suggestion of Carlo Urbani, an Italian physician working for the World Health Organization, who identified the first case of the disease outside China while treating patients in Vietnam and later passed away.

While further deliberation of the pathogenesis, and in fact, the mentioning of the atypical pneumonia itself, was withheld in the news media thereafter, the research community did not stop the exploration. In Beijing, China's capital, the Chinese Academy of Military Medical Sciences (CAMMS), an important medical research institution with the purview of fast response to any possible biological and chemical attack, took the disease seriously. With the approval from the Health Division under the People's Liberation Army (PLA) General Logistics Department, it dispatched the epidemiologist Cao Wuchun and the virologist Zhu Qingyu to the infection areas in Guangdong to collect specimen on the day following the Guangzhou press conference. Although they did receive some help from the PLA No. 1 Medical University, the PLA Guangzhou Military Region General Hospital, and Nanfang Hospital, they only got a thumb-sized lung tissue, some serum samples, and a few drops of saliva while in Guangzhou.[6]

In mid-February, a deputy director of the Institute of Virology under the China's national CDC brought from Guangzhou to Beijing two lung tissues from a deceased SARS patient, the portion reserved for it in the first Nanfang Hospital autopsy. The samples were then divided into three parts: one for Hong Tao, the CDC's chief virologist and also a CAE member, to conduct an electron microscope examination, one for the virologist Li Dexin to run the polymerase chain reaction (or PCR) testing, and the third for the bacterium cultivation purpose. Hong Tao soon found chlamydia, a bacterium notorious for being the cause of a common sexually transmitted disease but less fatal, on an electron microscopy and concluded that chlamydia was the pathogen of the atypical pneumonia. The Chinese CDC then held a press conference on February 18, during which the Director Li Liming announced Hong's discovery. Because Hong is an elite CAE member and authority of virology and possesses resources, the chlamydia hypothesis became the official line in China for the cause of the atypical pneumonia.

[6] Yan Xinhua and Zhang Ke. "Days and nights when Chinese scientists researched on the cause of SARS" (in Chinese), *People's Daily*, 18 Apr 2003; and interview (Beijing, China; 10 Nov 2003).

But some scientists, including those within the national CDC, and clinical physicians who had treated atypical pneumonia patients were skeptical of the finding. In Guangzhou, for example, doctors were strongly against Hong's theory and never treated patients in the protocol suggested by the national CDC. For Zhong Nanshan, to reach the chlamydia conclusion depending merely upon the morphological examination on an electron microscope is scientifically faulty; in order to determine a pathogen, he argued, one has to analyze the genetic characteristics, or the entire genetic sequence; the serum experiment is also important.[7] Clinical evidence also suggested that antibiotics against chlamydia had proven to be ineffective in treating the atypical pneumonia patients.

At the same time, in the CAMMS, the virologist Zhu Qingyu and his colleagues at the Institute of Microbiology and Epidemiology worked on the limited samples collected from Guangzhou. They grew the tissue samples in cell cultures and suckling mice and also took snapshots using an electron microscope. One of the images, taken on February 20, despite not clearly enough because of the low magnifying rate, showed that the virus has a distinctive halo of spikes that put it in a family not known to kill humans: the coronaviruses. By the first week of March, the group had tentative evidence that the new virus might indeed be linked to the epidemic. But the chlamydia hypothesis had become so well established that it would not have been respectful to challenge it and Hong Tao, Zhu's colleague Yang Ruifu said.[8] It was until March 21 after the CAMMS group collected more tissues from new cases in Beijing that linked the possible pathogen of the atypical pneumonia to coronavirus morphologically, and obtained the further evidence of the existence of coronavirus from serum epidemiology, immunology, and molecular biology did they report their definite finding to the PLA General Logistics Department and then the Ministry of Health (MOH) for approval. But if the finding had been announced immediately, it would still have been the first in the world.

[7] Liao Huailing. "The victory of the honesty".

[8] Martin Enserink. "China's missed chance"; He Shan and Zhu Xianghua. "Chinese scientists: We did not lose" (in Chinese), *Xin Bulletin*, 21 Jul 2003. According to the *Liberation Army Daily*, a PLA newspaper, the first virus image was taken on February 26. See Liu Yiqiang, Wu Zhijun and Liu Xingan. "The 66 days and nights in the fight against SARS" (in Chinese), *Liberation Army Daily*, 23 Apr 2003, p. 1.

While scientists around the world tackling the pathogen of SARS narrowed down the possibility to coronavirus, the "new, variant chlamydia" theory still dominated China. In a March 31 interview, Hong Tao indicated that although he could not rule out other possibilities, such as the "joint effects" of chlamydia and coronavirus, chlamydia is absolutely the main cause. In another press conference on April 4, China's national CDC Director Li Liming not only emphasized that Hong Tao found chlamydia-like agents through the interdisciplinary efforts of morphology, immunology, virology, and molecular biology, but also particularly mentioned: "When I indicated that we have had serum reaction in presenting our chlamydia finding to a World Health Organization (WHO) daily teleconference, the evidence was so powerful that no one challenged it." Even after the Chinese CDC informed the WHO that it also found the coronavirus, on April 12, Hong Tao still insisted his chlamydia-coronavirus coexistence theory. He further indicated that although China lagged behind the world in the coronavirus finding, it was the first country to identify chlamydia in SARS patients, and that chlamydia could be working in tandem with coronavirus. He even submitted a paper to the *Lancet* on April 13, suggesting the "synthetic roles" of chlamydia-like agents and the new coronavirus in the deadly respiratory illness.[9] Again, at this critical juncture, the Chinese CDC, or the so-called "national team" in Li Liming's words, gave the impression that China was on the right track to trace the cause of the atypical pneumonia.

When a public health crisis strikes, a country demands predicative and diagnostic certainty as quickly as possible. But because diseases are inherently complex, and their causes and courses are hard to foresee precisely, predictive and diagnostic failure (or, at least, delay) may occur.[10] That is what happened in the early stage of the AIDS epidemic when competing theories — some even ideologically based — were used to explain the cause of AIDS.[11] Likewise, immediately after SARS hit, scientists

[9] "Pressing ahead with SARS battle", *China Daily*, 15 Apr 2003.

[10] Christopher H. Foreman Jr. 1994. *Plague, Products, and Politics: Emergent Public Health Hazards and National Policymaking*. Washington, DC: The Brookings Institute, p. 27.

[11] Steven Epstein. 1996. *Impure Science: AIDS, Activism, and the Politics of Knowledge*. Berkeley, CA: University of California Press, pp. 45–178.

worldwide came up with various theories to explain the possible causes of the aliment. For example, Guangdong found from ten of the 41 patients' serum antibodies to gland virus, one of the common viruses that cause the respiratory infection; but its health officials made it clear that the finding was inconclusive until a comparison between the patients' serum during the infection and recovery periods is done. The WHO SARS network also produced varying, and at times, confusing, results, such as paramyxovirus, metapneumovirus, and pleiomorphic virus. However, in China, any challenge to the chlamydia theory was suppressed as institutionally any new finding was required to go through a clearinghouse — China's national CDC and the MOH, which until mid-April still covered up an SARS epidemic in China. Indeed, alternative explanations were effectively banned. The above-mentioned dissent views of Zhong Nanshan and his colleagues in Guangdong appeared in local newspapers, but did not become mainstream arguments. Bi Shengli, one of Hong Tao's colleagues at the Institute of Virology, found himself locked out because he disagreed with Hong of his conclusion about chlamydia and SARS. When Bi and Li Dexin, another Hong's colleague, broke the silence to announce their finding on the coronavirus through newspapers on April 11, they were criticized by Health Minister Zhang Wenkang for disrespecting the official conclusion and blocked further publication beyond.[12] Afterward, the MOH declared in the Chinese Central Television's prime-time news that any announcement of finding of the SARS pathogen without the approval of the MOH SARS Prevention and Treatment Leading Group is unofficial.[13]

China's national CDC, established in January 2002 on the Chinese Academy of Preventive Medicine, is to follow the model of the U.S. CDC. Although its facilities were not advanced and even shabby at the time of the SARS outbreak, the CDC occupied a very powerful and advantageous position. With the government's mandate, for example, hospitals around the country were required to hand in pathological samples from all SARS

[12] Charles Hutzler. "Chinese researchers' false start: Mistaken identity of germ culprit cost government time, prestige", *The Wall Street Journal*, 4 Jun 2003, pp. B1 and B3.

[13] Liao Huailing. "The victory of the honesty".

autopsies. But the center not only monopolized the dissemination of information on the disease — no individuals and institutions were allowed to announce research findings and publish papers without its consent, but also played "politics". In the case of the chlamydia controversy, it did not meet the requirement of the "Koch's postulates" in determining a disease-causing microorganism,[14] and later would be proved wrong, but the CDC defended it furiously, rather than attempting to replicate the result on which the assertion of fact was based or testing it in further studies and to seek consensus (or at least a modal position within a distribution of opinion), as a center for disease control and prevention is supposed to do.[15] Because of its misuse of the authority and power and the resulting resources allocated, China's CDC not only led researchers down a wrong path, but actually misled and hindered research on SARS. In efforts to save face and maintain its authority, the CDC damaged the credibility of Chinese scientists and cost dearly to Chinese citizens' lives.[16]

THE BEIJING GENOMICS INSTITUTE AND THE VIRUS GENOME SEQUENCING

As the above narrative indicates, between mid-February and mid-April, at least three groups of Chinese scientists were working on the pathogenesis of SARS — the Zhu Qingyu group at the CAMMS, the Hong Tao group and the Li Dexin and Bi Shengli group at the Chinese CDC. In the

[14] The "Koch's postulates", named after Robert Koch, the 19th-century German microbiologist, consist of four steps to prove the causation between a causal agent and an illness. First, the causal agent must be present in every case of the disease; second, it must be isolated from the host with the disease and grown in pure culture; third, the specific disease must be reproduced when a pure culture of the bacteria is inoculated into a healthy susceptible host; and fourth, the causal agent must be recoverable from the experimentally infected host. See http://www.medterms.com/script/main/art.asp?articlekey=7105, accessed on 20 Oct 2003.

[15] Christopher H. Foreman Jr. *Plague, Products, and Politics*, p. 53.

[16] Zhang Wenkang, then the health minister with training in medicine, presumably knew that chlamydia is no big deal, which explains why he dared to conceal the SARS outbreak (interview, Beijing, China; 3 Dec 2003).

meantime, a few Chinese biologists also tried to get the tissue samples from deceased patients, whose main interest was to sequence the genome of the SARS-causing virus. The following discussion will focus on one of the genome research powerhouses in the world — the Beijing Genomics Institute (BGI).

The BGI was a product of China's participation in the International Human Genome Project (IHGP), the interests of a group of Chinese life scientists working overseas, including Yang Huanming and Wang Jian, to contribute to their motherland, and the efforts of the Chinese Academy of Sciences (CAS) to build the academy into a world-class research establishment. With the support from the CAS, a Human Genome Center (HGC) was first set up within the CAS Institute of Genetics, which evolved into the BGI formally in July 1999. Two months later, during the fifth conference on the strategy discussion of the IHGP in London, Yang Huanming reported the preparative work done at the BGI on the participation of the IHGP, and then the BGI was officially accepted to the consortium and allocated the task of sequencing 1% of the human genome. Later, China's Ministry of Science and Technology (MOST) and the CAS also jumped on the bandwagon and turned the 1% project to a national research priority. The BGI, along with China's National Human Genome Centers in Beijing and Shanghai, completed the work in April 2000. From then on, the BGI has been also involved in other high-profile genome-sequencing projects, such as the super hybrid rice (*indica*) genome and the porcine genome. It is fair to say that as one of the world's most advanced sequencing and genomics research centers, the BGI is capable of producing first-rate work and playing an important role in cracking the genome of the SARS virus. In fact, the British Columbia Cancer Agency Genome Sciences Center in Vancouver, Canada, which, according to Wang Jian, executive director of the BGI, who used to be in charge of the technical work in that center, is much smaller than the BGI in scale, won the competition in sequencing the genome of the SARS virus. It is against this backdrop that Yang Huanming made the sober claim: "Chinese scientists were defeated by SARS."

If China's failure to first identify the pathogen of SARS is mainly due to the misuse of power and authority by Hong Tao and China's national CDC, the BGI lost the virus genome sequencing battle because it did not have the virus materials to work with. There was guess that the BGI might just not be interested in such "*toufu*-type" work (the coronavirus has 29,736 pairs of nucleotides, compared with the rice genome's more than 400 million pairs), while at that time it had several multi-million dollar projects running. There was also suspicion that only when China's political leadership took step to ease the crisis did the BGI start to publicize itself, which explains why the institute posted in GenBank partial sequences of five isolates with minimal fanfare to avoid offending authorities and Yang Huanming had kept low-profile until President Hu Jintao's visit to the BGI, a contradiction to his personality.[17]

According to Chinese news reports, upon learning the outbreak of a mysterious and deadly pneumonia, Wang Jian realized the urgency and value of sequencing the virus genome. He had been to the infection areas in Guangdong three times and later hospitals in Beijing in search of virus samples, but returned empty handed. In one occasion, he was bluntly told: "Why should I give you the samples that we gathered from the 'forefront' (*qianxian*) with the danger of losing our lives? We would rather throw the samples away even if we could not get anything from them."[18] The news reports went on to say that Wang and his colleagues had to sneak into a Beijing hospital to "steal" samples. In order not to be recognized, they wore hats and masks and got in between 10 pm and 7 am. But Chen Hao, who was then with the CAS Bureau of Science Policy and later appointed deputy director of the BGI, indicated that Chinese scientists are accustomed to waiting for tasks and seeking funding for mid- and long-term programs, rather than taking initiatives on emergent projects. Accordingly, when SARS struck, few acted until President Hu spoke out.[19] Finally, the BGI did get some tissue samples on April 9; but without expertise in virus isolation and cultivation, it was unable to produce genome sequences immediately.[20]

[17] Dennis Normile. "Hungry for details, scientists zoom in on SARS genomes", *Science*, Vol. 300 (2 May 2003), pp. 715–716.

[18] See http://chanye.sina.net/yy/2003-06-12/169793.shtml, accessed on 12 Jul 2003.

[19] Xie Xiang and Zhu Xinyu. "Yang Huanming's pain".

[20] Interview (Beijing, China; 10 Nov 2003).

In retrospect, tissue samples from SARS patients became a precious commodity so that many scientists and institutions would like to obtain them. China's national CDC, by law, is the possessor of virus samples. Nevertheless, even virologists at China's national CDC complained of not having enough materials to work with.[21] Despite having connections in Guangdong, the CAMMS scientists did not get much of what they wanted when they returned from the field such that one of the scientists cried at the Guangzhou airport, feeling the mission unaccomplished.

In the meantime, many owners of the tissues did not have the capability to handle the virus. Back then, the CAMMS was the only institution that had a truly Class III pathogen lab, one with the highest biosafety. But the CAMMS group did not necessarily make the best use of the tissue samples either. Although it obtained the first electron microscope image of the possible coronavirus on February 20, the first in the world, the scientists seemed not to think of working with others; even when they reported the definite finding to the PLA General Logistics Department and the MOH on March 21, the CAMMS still wanted to do the virus genome sequencing on their own, an area that the institution apparently does not have the expertise. It later decided to seek help from the BGI on the virus genome sequencing for two probable reasons: first, to speed up the research so as to meet the recently increasing attention to the aliment by the political leadership; and second, to weather the mounting pressure that a delay would be politicized. An agreement was thus reached at 6 pm on April 15, which stipulates that the virus samples be delivered to the BGI by midnight of that day. Although it took the BGI 36 hours to sequence the genomes of four viral strains, it was too late for both the BGI and the CAMMS to receive their due credit and claim priority, because the Canadian group had already put the coronavirus genome sequence on its website two days ago.[22]

But clinical physicians contested the accusation of their being uncooperative in providing virus samples for the pathological examination

[21] Charles Hutzler. "Chinese researchers' false start".

[22] Yan Xinhua and Zhang Ke. "Days and nights when Chinese scientists researched on the cause of SARS". However, one would also wonder why the BGI did not contact the CAMMS as soon as it got tissue samples.

and genome sequencing efforts. "They just did not approach us," said Zhong Nanshan, the Guangzhou doctor. However, at the request of scientists from Hong Kong, Zhong started in the end of February to share the tissues with them, including the virologist Malik Peiris at the University of Hong Kong (HKU) who would become widely recognized for finding that the coronavirus causes SARS. In fact, upon hearing the rumors of an unusual outbreak of severe pneumonia in Guangdong in January, Peiris had kept an eye on that and collaborated with physicians in Guangdong.[23]

The international life science labs used to fight fiercely to be the first to finger a culprit and sharing data or samples was often out of the question. But this time, a global network of labs has largely survived the furious rivalries traditionally dominating the competitive field of virology. When epidemiologically linked clusters of SARS cases began to spread from China through Hong Kong to the world, under the coordination of the WHO, scientists around the world built a global SARS research network and nurtured an atmosphere in which normal scientific competition could be somewhat suspended. The WHO issued its global SARS alert on March 12, and by March 17, Dr. Klaus Stöhr, a German-born virologist who leads the WHO's Global Influenza Surveillance Network, invited eleven labs — in Atlanta, Winnipeg, London, Paris, Frankfurt, Rotterdam, Tokyo, Singapore, and Hong Kong — to participate in a coordinated worldwide scientific onslaught on the epidemic.[24] This virtual laboratory launched a global-spanning team effort dedicated to finding the cause of SARS as fast as possible. It held daily teleconferences to share findings with each other, and posted genetic sequences, electron

[23] Liao Huailing. "The victory of honesty".

[24] World Health Organization Multicenter Collaborative Network for Severe Acute Respiratory Syndrome (SARS) Diagnosis. "A multicenter collaboration to investigate the cause of severe acute respiratory syndrome", *Lancet*, Vol. 361 (17 May 2003), pp. 1730–1733. It is unknown why the Beijing and Guangdong labs were not invited at the beginning, although they joined the network on March 28. Dr. Stöhr has not responded to the author's e-mail inquiries; he quitted his position as SARS research coordinator in part because he did not receive enough support from the WHO. See Martin Enserink and Dennis Normile. "Search for SARS origins stalls", *Science*, Vol. 302 (31 Oct 2003), pp. 766–767.

microscope images, and other data on a secure Web site. Reagents were shipped around the world within hours of a collaborator's request. The "historic" collaboration speeded up the hunting for the culprit "two or three times faster", as one of the participants indicated.[25]

The first hints about the probable culprit came on March 21, just four days after the formation of the network, when the virologist Peiris of the HKU e-mailed group members that he had isolated a virus from patient tissues. It grew more slowly when exposed to serum from patients recovering from a SARS infection, suggesting they had developed antibodies to the virus. Serum from healthy controls had no effect on the virus. An initial electron microscope image suggested a coronavirus.[26]

The findings were replicated in other labs, and on March 24, Julie Gerberding, director of the U.S. CDC in Atlanta, announced the American finding of the coronavirus to the world.[27] On April 13, Canadian scientists finished the sequencing of the genome of the susceptible coronavirus related to SARS. Immediately followed were similar genomes sequenced by the U.S. CDC, the CAMMS and the BGI, and the HKU. On April 15, the WHO announced in Geneva that a novel variety of the coronavirus is the pathogen that causes SARS, which settles the competition for priority in the hunting. The next day, Dutch scientists in the WHO network announced confirmation that SARS is caused by the highly susceptible coronavirus through the experiment on African green monkey — the final procedure of the "Koch's postulates". Two weeks later, two papers on the SARS virus genomes — one by the Canadian scientists and the other by a joint team between the U.S. CDC and the University of California at San Francisco — were immediately referred and posted at the website of *Science*, one of the leading international scientific journals. "Both research teams produced these

[25] Martin Enserink and Gretchen Vogel. "Deferring competition, global net closes in on SARS", *Science*, Vol. 300 (11 Apr 2003), pp. 224–225.

[26] Dennis Normile. "Up close and personal with SARS", *Science*, Vol. 300 (9 May 2003), pp. 886–887.

[27] Martin Enserink and Gretchen Vogel. "Deferring competition, global net closes in on SARS".

genomic sequences quickly and efficiently, in a model of cooperation among various groups," said *Science*'s Editor-in-Chief Don Kennedy.[28]

Historically, Chinese scientists from different jurisdictions had worked together on important, government-initiated projects and successfully executed them, the achievements of the strategic weapons (the so-called *liangdan yixing*) program and the most recent *Shenzhou* manned spaceflight program being two examples. One of the characteristics of such efforts is the organizational style of "competitive horizontalism", or the collaboration across fragmented vertical bureaucratic hierarchies.[29] In the mid-1980s, China started to reform its science and technology management system to strengthen the link not only between the research community and the economy but also between different administrative jurisdictions. The mechanism through which the nation's scientific activities are coordinated was the Leading Group on Science and Technology in 1983, renamed the Leading Group on Science, Technology, and Education in 1998, in the State Council.[30] However, too many bureaucratic fiefdoms have been struggling with each other over political and economic interests and dispensing scarce resources on frequently redundant research programs with competing priorities, which, coupled with clashes over control of one's turf, has resulted in ineffective spending in research and development.

When SARS struck, scientists from China's civilian and military medical research establishments knew the importance of getting involved and where their focus should be from their own interests. For the CAMMS, detecting the pathogen associated to SARS might be a good exercise for handling possible biological and chemical attacks in the future, although it ruled out the possibility of a man-made culprit at the

[28] http://www.aaas.org/news/releases/2003/0501sars.shtml, accessed on 2 May 2003.

[29] Evan A. Feigenbaum. 2003. *China's Techno-Warriors: National Security and Strategic Competition from the Nuclear to the Information Age*. Stanford, CA: Stanford University Press, pp. 39–60.

[30] Tony Saich. 1989. *China's Science Policy in the 80s*. Atlantic Highlands, NJ: Humanities Press International, pp. 60–66; Richard P. Suttmeier and Cong Cao. "China faces the new industrial revolution: Assessing research and innovation strategies for the 21st century", *Asian Perspective*, Vol. 24, No. 3 (1999), pp. 153–200.

very beginning;[31] sequencing the SARS virus genome might earn the BGI high publicity; and medical doctors might like to share with established partners to get their credit. Also at stake were the potential economic payoffs from the research. But researchers were not necessarily willing to collaborate with each other. To meet the requirement of the "Koch's postulates", for example, the Guangdong CDC did three verifications of the coronavirus, but not the fourth one — an animal experiment because of the unavailability of the facility. On April 2, its virologist Yan Xinge brought a culture sample to the national CDC for help. But the experts in Beijing would rather possess the virus sample and run the entire testing themselves than working with the Guangdong group.[32] Therefore, China's failure to first identify the coronavirus and sequence its genome, simply put, was also due to the organizational obstacles that hindered collaboration and the malfunction of coordination among different institutions from the scientific leadership.

Publication and the Advance of Knowledge

The Chinese scientific and medical community seems to disagree with Yang Huanming's sensational argument that Chinese scientists were defeated by SARS. One piece of evidence they would present is China's low mortality rate among SARS patients. According to the WHO statistics, the cumulative mortality rate related to SARS is 9.6%, but would be significantly high at 15.3% if not the low mortality rate in China, which is only 6.5%, were excluded (Table 1). The statistics seem to suggest that China has been quite successful in treating SARS patients at the clinical level, which has in turn made significant contributions to the reduction of death from the disease worldwide.[33] In other words, the cumulative

[31] Qin E'de. *et al.* "A complete sequence and comparative analysis of a SARS-associated virus (Isolate BJ01)", *Chinese Science Bulletin*, Vol. 48, No. 10 (2003), pp. 941–948.

[32] Li Yuanli. "Why did China lose in the SARS research?" (in Chinese), *China Business News*, 9 Jun 2003.

[33] Ironically, the success in containing SARS was a consequence of rigorous international efforts in isolating infected people.

Table 1. Cumulative Number of Reported Probable Cases of SARS

Country	Cumulative number of cases	Number of deaths	Cumulative mortality rate (%)
China, Taiwan	346	37	10.7
China, Hong Kong SAR	1755	299	17.0
Singapore	238	33	13.9
Canada	251	43	17.1
World Total	8098	774	9.6
China	**5327**	**349**	**6.5**
World Total, China excluded	2771	425	15.3

Source: World Health Organization, http://www.who.int/csr/sars/country/table2003_09_23/en/, accessed on 22 Dec 2003.

mortality of the SARS patients could be significantly reduced if the Chinese experience had been shared internationally immediately.

One may argue that the lower death rate among SARS patients in China may have something to do with the characteristics of the virus itself or the gene of Chinese, in addition to the conventional wisdom that the Chinese statistics were not trustworthy.[34] But according to Zhong Nanshan, one of the first physicians at the forefront of diagnosing and treating SARS patients, the low mortality rate among Chinese SARS patients could be attributed to two factors. First, China concentrated patients needed critical care in a few designated hospitals with well-trained doctors, better treatment facilities, and combined efforts of respiratory, intensive care, and infectious disease units. The hospital in Xiaotangshan, a suburb of Beijing, was set up and staffed in six days for that purpose. Second, Chinese doctors have adopted a comprehensive treatment protocol which included the appropriate use of corticosteroids and BiPAP, a non-invasive pressure ventilation method, and the combined therapy of traditional Chinese medicine and Western medicine.

[34] Chinese statistics has always had the problem of underreport or overreport. In the case of SARS, between November 2002 and mid-April 2003, the outbreak was covered up.

In order to convince and help their foreign peers, Chinese physicians are supposed to take quick action to get their results published. Because lives are at stake, the international journals have taken measures to expedite the review and publication process and to disseminate information through the Internet before the formal publication of papers. For example, Canadian scientists produced the SARS virus genome sequence on April 13, and submitted a paper to *Science* two days later; the paper was online on May 1 along with another paper by American scientists. Zhong Nanshan himself had a similar experience. He was invited to the American Thoracic Society (ATS) 2003 amid the global SARS crisis. His paper based on the May 18 presentation was submitted on May 22 and accepted in final form by the *American Journal of Respiratory Critical Care Medicine* within 24 hours, and put online on May 28.[35]

Although Chinese doctors might have successfully figured out and used effective treatment protocols, their clinical efforts have been mostly unknown to the international medical community, because physicians in the mainland have thus far failed to have their papers on the treatment published in leading international journals. Again, according to Zhong Nanshan, Chinese doctors did not have time to write papers while they were busy treating patients; or further, they lacked the mindset of timely summarizing their experience and publishing papers, different from their basic research peers who are eager to get into the publication game.[36] As a whole, of the papers published in *Science*, *Nature*, *Lancet*, the *New England Journal of Medicine*, the *Journal of American Medical Association*, few belong to scientists and physicians from mainland China. That is, they were defeated on another front.[37]

Withholding successful treatment protocols is a violation of the norms of scientific and medical professions, if not immoral, given that

[35] Zhong Nanshan and Zeng Guangqiao. "Our strategies for fighting severe acute respiratory syndrome (SARS)", *American Journal of Respiratory Care Medicine*, Vol. 168 (1 Jul 2003), pp. 7–9.

[36] One may say that physicians as well as lawyers have different incentives from their basic scientists.

[37] That situation has gradually changed as Chinese scientists published several important papers in the *Proceeding of the National Academy of Sciences* and *Science* in late 2003.

SARS is expected to come back and even become a common infectious disease. The question is whether Chinese doctors do have something special to offer. In this regard, the Zhong Nanshan case is suggestive. His ATS presentation, mentioned above, on the appropriate use of corticosteroids and BiPAP was anecdotal such that he did not convince the conference participants as to why the endeavors of his and his colleagues worked as indicated. In revising the paper, he added the role of the traditional Chinese medicine but did not give many details. Zhong proposed that the recovery of patients from SARS depends upon their immune systems, but seemed to have difficulty reconciling this with the fact that the use of steroids in a large dosage in fact could suppress the immune systems. Similarly, the Chinese news media praised Dr. Jiang Suchun, an infectious-disease expert at the PLA No. 302 Hospital, who became infected with SARS soon after he began treating patients, for using himself as a guinea pig: he injected serum from recovered SARS patients and got well after 23 days;[38] but how effective was this treatment method when applied to a larger patient population? There are news reports on the effective role that the traditional Chinese medicine has played in treating SARS patients;[39] again, what are the data to support this claim?

Until recently, traditional Chinese medicine is not subjected to controlled trials as it was employed by historical precedent.[40] But modern medicine is no longer based on experience; instead, it is a science that involves theory-directed treatment protocols established through research design, step-by-step controlled trials, analysis of the treatment results, and the combined efforts of basic scientists and clinical practitioners. Although Chinese scientists may have accumulated experience

[38] *Liberation Army Daily*, 25 Apr 2003, p. 1.

[39] See, for example, http://www.sars.ac.cn/shwo.phd?id=5756, accessed on 16 Jul 2003; http://www.sars.ac.cn/shwo.phd?id=7130, http://www.sars.ac.cn/shwo.phd?id=7132, http://www.sars.ac.cn/shwo.phd?id=7134, accessed on 28 Jul 2003; http://www.peopledaily.com.cn/GB/shehui/212/10548/10649/1949890.html, http://www.peopledaily.com.cn/GB/shizheng/19/20030609/1012877.html, accessed on 18 Jul 2003, *Science Times*, 9 Oct 2003.

[40] Gail E. Henderson and Myron S. Cohen. 1984. *The Chinese Hospital: A Socialist Work Unit*. New Haven, CT: Yale University Press, p. 132.

through diagnosing and treating many SARS patients, and have successfully combined traditional Chinese medicine with Western medicine, until they put the experience in the perspective of modern medicine, what they have done is at the experience level as traditional Chinese medicine has been in the course of several thousand years. That is, it is unsystematic, lacking modern scientific basis, and depending upon the trial-and-error method. This is exactly the pitfall that Zhong Nanshan's paper published in the *American Journal of Respiratory Critical Care Medicine* suffered, which, along with the contradiction between the use of corticosteroids and the role of immune systems, may explains why the paper was published as an occasional essay, a category lower than a formal paper.[41]

As the analysis goes, it is more likely that the Chinese medical community has not seriously looked into the data and come up with convincing theories despite having more than 5,000 cases of SARS and 349 deaths. Chinese doctors have not advanced medical knowledge in the course of fighting against SARS. Therefore, the low mortality rate reported for Chinese SARS patients would become skeptical.

Post-Crisis Efforts and Persistent Problems

In mid-April, when the international pressure accumulated, China's political leadership started to take note. The Party General Secretary Hu Jintao inspected the Guangdong CDC and the Premier Wen Jiabao convened a State Council meeting to discuss the establishment of a national mechanism to deal with the public health emergency. On April 20, China finally lifted the restriction on the publicity of SARS, removed the health minister and the Beijing mayor from their positions for their inability in handling the crisis, and mandated further sanctions to those who failed to report the SARS cases. On the same day, President Hu inspected the CAMMS and the BGI, boosting the morale of the

[41] Xiao Qiao. "SARS in China", http://www.xys.org/xys/ebooks/others/science/misc/sars_jinian.txt, accessed on 23 Aug 2003.

scientists at the frontier of the SARS research. In the meantime, as the epidemic spread, attracted more press coverage, and generated more effective lobbying from the scientific and medical community, the commitment to the aliment ballooned.

China's rigid science and technology system is partly to blame for having not responded to the SARS crisis quickly and effectively; that system has not changed in the post-crisis environment. The difference is that it has just gone to the other extreme: each institution, regardless of its capability and expertise, wants to conduct SARS-related research. China's scientific leadership has ever since made moves to support the SARS research, especially on the search of vaccines that would permanently dismantle the disease. But there is still no coordination of research efforts at different jurisdictions so that there could be enormous waste of human and financial resources.

First, by taking advantage of the nation's new priority — the war on SARS, the scientific and medical community has requested and received an increased amount of funding. But in many instances, the funding decisions were made through *ad libitum* way and unprecedented rapidity. For example, while inspecting the CAMMS on April 19, the Chief of the PLA General Logistics Department Liao Xilong approved an expenditure of RMB10 million to the academy on site.[42] Later, the SARS Research Leading Group funded 95 research projects with a combined expenditure of RMB120 million.[43] Probably out of the considerations to balance the interests of different jurisdictions — national and local, civilian and military, universities and research institutes, the funding intensity was too low for serious research. The total expenditure for the 61 projects funded by the National Natural Science Foundation of China (NSFC), for example, was RMB10.25 million, with an average of RMB170,000 (Table 2). The peer review mechanism was sacrificed in the name of speeding up the process, even in the NSFC that has had a good reputation of supporting the best research in China through fair competition and rigorous review. One awardee indicated that it was a matter of days between the proposal

[42] *People's Daily*, 18 May 2003, p. 1.

[43] *Science Times*, 1 Aug 2003.

Table 2. Funding of SARS-Related Projects at the National Natural Science Foundation of China

Academic division	Number of projects	Total funds (RMB, million)	Average funds per project (RMB)
Life Science	22	6	272727
Chemistry	8	1.05	131250
Earth Science	2	0.9	450000
Engineering and Material Science	13	1.3	100000
Management Science	16	1	62500
Total	61	10.25	168033

Source: National Natural Science Foundation of China, http://www.nsfc.gov.cn/nsfc/cen/sars/news/news15.htm, accessed on 17 Jul 2003.

submission and the money distribution.[44] One consequence of the increased funding is the rush to set up Class III pathogen labs. In addition to the cost of millions for the construction of each of them, there are concerns such as whether other capabilities for such labs, especially personnel, are available, whether these labs will be efficiently utilized, and whether they themselves meet the WHO lab safety guidelines so as not to cause the leak of toxic materials and infection of those who do research inside.[45]

Second, because of the visibility of the SARS research and subsequent institutional support and engagement, there has been a new "great leap forward". Researchers have announced one achievement after another through the news media with the focus on the advancement in the SARS vaccines. Although many of the announcements were made by institutions not capable of conducting such research and the "science through news conference" that do not provide the necessary scientific information is unacceptable to the scientific community, this practice itself shows a tendency of pursuing quick and immediate results that has

44 Zhang Jing. "SARS attacked China's research management system".

45 See http://www.ycwb.com/gb/content/2003-07/21/content_556460.htm, accessed on 22 Jul 2003; David Cyranoski. "SARS triggers biomedical shake-up in China", *Nature*, Vol. 25 (25 Sept 2003), p. 333. The recent lab accidents or cases of contamination in Singapore and Taiwan sound the alarm to China.

prevailed in the Chinese scientific community in the recent decade. The irony is that researchers working on SARS have to depend upon Chinese media accounts to know what their peers are doing.[46] In the meantime, there still lacks serious research to pin down the source of the infection, or the index animals that harbor the virus. In fact, this kind of research — whether SARS make a simple leap from such animals as civet straight to humans or did the virus travel through some other species first — is more arduous to conduct, but more fundamental in answering how coronavirus has been transmitted from animals to human beings as SARS is a zoonotic epidemic.

Third, in light of the crisis and the lack of coordination, a group of scientists involved in biomedical research has called for the establishment of a Chinese version of the National Institutes of Health (NIH),[47] which means resources reallocation and mobilization. While the suggestion of founding such an institution and having stable support has its merit, at issue are probably the accountability and the better utilization of the existing institutions and their current concrete and feasible response to the novel situation rather than another agency with bureaucratic power.

Fourth, also in the face of persistent funding constraint in China, there is always the question of "who spends how much on what", this time the situation may be getting even worse. That is, the scale of the increases may prompt claims whether the SARS research has received funding at the level that does not necessarily commensurate with the seriousness of the illness, that is, it may have begun to swallow too large a slice of the funding pie. And because cancer, heart diseases, and AIDS, among others, have claimed more lives than SARS in China, diverting resources to SARS means the relative neglect of these more urgent illnesses.

CONCLUSION

Although SARS occurred first in China which also had the most cases, scientists and physicians from mainland China have failed to capitalize

[46] Lawrence K. Altman. "China lags in sharing SARS clues, officials say", *The New York Times*, 5 Aug 2003.

[47] David Cyranoski. "SARS triggers biomedical shake-up in China".

on their advantages and resources. The SARS outbreak has revealed serious shortcomings of the China scientific and medical community to respond to emerging diseases. Were these the problems of individual scientists, of institutions, or of culture?

Although science is competitive in nature, it could become cooperative, especially when parties involved could tackle a problem quickly through the division of labor, or from different perspectives, when scientists in a nation work together amid international competition, and when there is an emergency that calls for the combined endeavor of the scientific community. This time, China's scientists could definitely turn the SARS crisis to an opportunity to show off their growing scientific prowess. But the scientific leadership was incapable of taking initiatives to coordinate the activities across different jurisdictions; as a result, the orchestrated efforts did not exist while resources and personnel mobilization — one of the legacies of the communist regime — encountered its worst nightmare. Therefore, on the surface, it is the Chinese scientists who lost in the international competition for priority; but it is essentially more a failure of China's science system, for which unfortunately its leadership has not acknowledged its inability and ineffectiveness and accepted its responsibility.[48]

Behaviorally, scientists are guided by a set of norms, one of which is to have an organized or conditioned skepticism toward existing knowledge and challenge the false claims regardless of the status of those who propose them.[49] However, because of the so-called "Matthew effect", prestigious scientists tend to be more influential, not only in that they take credits inappropriately, but also in that challenging their wrong theories becomes more difficult, if not impossible.[50] That is what happened to the

[48] Xu Guanhua, China's science minister, for example, gave a score of 100 to Chinese scientists when asked to evaluate their performance in the fight against SARS in the China Central Television "Dialogue" program on 22 Jun 2003. See http://www.cctv.com.financial/20030623/100401.shtml, accessed on 12 Dec 2003.

[49] Robert K. Merton. 1973 (originally 1942). "The normative structure of science", in Robert K. Merton (Norman W. Storer [ed.]), *The Sociology of Science: Theoretical and Empirical Investigations*. Chicago, IL: University of Chicago Press, pp. 267–278.

[50] Robert K. Merton. (originally 1968). "The Matthew effect in science", in Merton, *The Sociology of Science* pp. 439–459.

chlamydia hypothesis. The theory was put forward by Hong Tao, an elite CAE member who stubbornly clung to the chlamydia theory. In addition, the Chinese CDC, which has acquired absolute authority through the government's mandate, shut out the arguments from clinicians and hampered the possibility to present alternative explanations by misusing, if not abusing, its institutional power. Under these circumstances, researchers at the CAMMS at least had to take a more careful and cautious attitude in offering their alternative hypothesis and challenging Hong Tao and the Chinese CDC.[51] These, plus the constraints placed on the CAMMS as a military scientific institution, prevented China from becoming the first country to claim that the coronavirus causes SARS.

Scientists mainly establish themselves through communicating new knowledge. In doing so, they give their "gift" to the community and receive or increase their credibility as return.[52] In the fight against SARS, Chinese scientists and physicians may have done first-rate work in research and patient treatment, but they were unable to participate in the international scholarly communication by publishing their research on a timely fashion. It is quite unfortunate that major findings in the SARS research were achieved by scientists from the countries that did not have many patients. Consequently, efforts by the Chinese scientific and medical community have been undermined; and scientists from outside China even cast doubt about the validity of China's low death rate among SARS patients.

Now, SARS is contained in China and scientists are enjoying increased funding and support. However, the scientific community and especially its leadership have not learned the lesson from their failures in the SARS crisis and taken concrete measures to improve the nation's research system. Independence is still the style characteristic of the behavior of many Chinese scientists. Will they be defeated a second time? The question is as serious today as it was a year ago.

[51] Interview (Beijing, China; 10 Nov 2003).

[52] Warren O. Hagstrom. 1965. *The Scientific Community*. New York: Basic Books, pp. 13–24; and Bruno Latour and Steve Walgar. 1986. *Laboratory Life: The Construction of Scientific Facts*. Princeton, NJ: Princeton University Press.

Chapter 7

SARS and Freedom of the Press: Has the Chinese Government Learnt a Lesson?

HE BAOGANG

In this age of information, it is a wonder why thousands of ordinary Chinese were not aware of the outbreak of SARS in March 2003. When SARS became the hottest issue in newspapers, radios, television and daily chats in Hong Kong and Singapore in February and March 2003, calls to Chinese relatives and friends in China about SARS met with surprising ignorance. This phenomenon is a reflection of a fundamental problem in the Chinese political system and its management of information.

SARS is an acronym for severe acute respiratory syndrome, a natural disease. However, this natural disease was worsened by a political SARS, that is "scandal authoritarian regime syndrome" in which the Chinese authoritarian politics operates through a system of controlling, hiding, distorting, and manipulating information about the SARS epidemic.

CHINESE AUTHORITARIANISM AND INFORMATION CONTROL SYSTEM

The mass media is a pillar of the Chinese authoritarian regime, and it is a device for inhibiting citizens against the regime. The media has supported and advanced the powers and policies of the authoritarian government. It is the nature of authoritarian government to control information. Information is the foundation on which an authoritarian government maintains its power and order. An authoritarian system often creates asymmetric information system, that is, top leaders have access to abundant information while ordinary people are provided with little information. This asymmetric information system provides an opportunity for bureaucrats to lie without being noticed, and to "sell" information for their material benefits.

China is not devoid of a mass communications system. By the end of 2002, China had 2,137 newspapers, 9,029 journals, 306 radio stations, 368 television stations, 1,526 wire broadcasting and television stations at county level, and 568 publishing houses. It is amazing thus that except for a few days in February 2003, there was no report on SARS during the early stages of the outbreak despite such a gigantic network of newspapers, journals, radios and television stations. The Party-State was so powerful that it was able to tighten up its control over the media through the following mechanisms and measures in 2002 when China was evaluated by Freedom House as "not free" country (see Table 1).

Holding conferences and training programs to unify ideas and actions. The National Propaganda Ministers' Conference and the National

Table 1. Comparative Measures of Freedom (Selected Countries)

Country	Political rights	Civil liberties	Freedom rating
Cambodia	6	5	Not Free
China (PRC)	**7**	**6**	**Not Free**
India*	2	3	Free
Japan*	1	2	Free
Korea, South*	2	2	Free
Malaysia	5	5	Partly Free
Philippines*	2	3	Free
Russia*	5	5	Partly Free
Singapore	5	5	Partly Free
Sri Lanka*	3	4	Partly Free
Taiwan (Rep. Of China)*	1	2	Free

Source: *Journal of Democracy*, Volume 13, No.1 (January 2002), pp. 108–109, modified.

Notes: *Indicates countries which are electoral democracies. The Freedom Rating is an overall judgment based on survey results.

Conference of Press and Publication Bureau Directors were held in January 2002, and over 600 chief editors were trained in 2002.

Institutionalize the domination of party newspapers. Party newspapers have been well established and supported at the national, provincial and city levels. To supplement this three-tier party newspapers system, the applications of 168 party newspapers at the prefecture city level were approved by General Administration of Press and Publication in 2002.[1]

Issuing certificate for job appointment. All directors, managers, and chief editors of presses, newspapers and journals must have official approved certificates for their appointment. They receive official orders from the Department of Propaganda on a regular basis. If they go beyond the confines of official lines, the certificates of the directors or chief editors of the newspapers and journals might be revoked, meaning that they will lose their jobs. The General Administration of Press and Publication issued the certificates in 2002 and would re-examine them every year.[2] Through the certificate control mechanism, the Department of Propaganda hoped that self-censorship will work. As Perry Link points out: "Questions of risk — how far to go, how explicit to be, with whom to ally, and so on — are moved inside the cerebrums of every individual writer and editor. There are, of course, physical punishments that anchor one's calculations. If you calculate incorrectly and go too far, you can lose your job, be imprisoned, or, in the worse case, get a bullet in the back of the head."[3]

Granting licenses: The General Administration of Press and Publication granted the licences for 13 media conglomerates (syndicates) in June and December 2002. It limits the maximum number of press conglomerates to no more than 50 by the end of 2004.[4] These conglomerates are organized to follow a line of Party media organs in order to ensure the Party's control over the media. Their activities cannot cross provincial

[1] *Zhongguo Chuban Nianjian 2003*. Beijing: Zhongguo chuban nianjianshe, 2003, p. 107.
[2] *Zhongguo Chuban Nianjian 2003*, p. 107.
[3] Perry Link. "The anaconda in the chandelier: Censorship in China today", *Asia Program Special Report*, Woodrow Wilson International Center for Scholars, No. 102, Apr 2002, p. 4.
[4] *Zhongguo Chuban Nianjian 2003*, p. 107.

borders and they can only operate printed media and not permitted to own any broadcasting institutions.[5]

Censorship system. To ensure "political correctness", a three-tier hierarchal censorship system was established in Hebei Province. At the lower level, the agency of each newspaper and journal will form a special reading group whose responsibility is to read and evaluate all incoming materials and to ensure conformity with the Party's propaganda agenda. At the middle level, 16 "readers" are appointed and paid by the Department of Propaganda to read and evaluate journals and newspapers as well as to publish bulletins. At the higher level, six "readers" from the division of newspaper and journal in the Department of News and Publisher, hold a weekly evaluation meeting to assess all newspapers and journals.[6]

"Saohuang" and "dafei" campaign. From June to December 2002 a national campaign "to clean up the media" was carried out. "*Saohuang*" aims to sweep away pornographic books and periodicals, and "*dafei*" cracks down on "illegal" political publications. In Beijing a special task force was established to eliminate all illegal political publications. The specific task was to ensure that within one hundred days before the 16th Party Congress, no newspaper and journal publishes anything on "illegal" political matter, no printing house prints anything that contains "illegal" political publications, and no bookstore sells any publication that contains "illegal" political matter. From August 23–25, 2002, the General Administration of Press and Publication sent an investigation team to Guangzhou and Shenzhen to assess the effectiveness of the "Saohuang" and "Dafei" campaign. It concluded that "illegal" political publications were eliminated in Guangzhou. A symposium on Press and Publication in Eastern Area was also held in Guangzhou from December 4–5, 2002.[7]

Management and "rectification" of newspapers and periodicals. Seventy newspapers and 48 journals (among them 36 are social sciences journals) were investigated and prosecuted in 2002. For newspapers, the license of

[5] Chin-Chuan Lee. "When power marries money: Media freedom in China", *Asia Program Special Report*, Woodrow Wilson International Center for Scholars, No. 102, Apr 2002, p. 15.

[6] *Zhongguo Chuban Nianjian 2003*, p. 109.

[7] *Ibid.*, pp. 51–62.

Special Economic Zone Time was revoked; the license of *City Economic Newspaper* was suspended; ten newspapers received "administrative warning", and 54 newspapers received the official notice for "breaking rules and regulations". For journals, the licenses of five journals were suspended; five journals were fined, 11 journals received "administrative warning", and 13 journals received official notice for "breaking rules and regulations". *Zhuyi Evening News* was criticized in the circulated official document for its report on the airplane clash in Hainan in 2001. One college journal received an official criticism for discussing the "one country and two systems" policy. *Zhongqing Commercial Newspaper* received an official notice or warning for breaking rules and regulations; that is, it downloaded a news piece about potential earthquake in Tibet from China's Daily Network and published it openly.[8]

Cyber censorship. Shanthi Kalathil and Taylor C. Boas argue that authoritarian governments, far from fearing the information age, have chosen to direct Internet development in ways that bolster the state.[9] In China, the Ministry of Public Security and the Ministry of Information Industry allotted sizeable financial and human resources to develop a secret "Golden Shield" program that employs a cyber police force of some 30,000 persons to spot, identify, and arrest dissident Internet users. The government has also issued more than 60 laws and regulations to control the Internet. For example, Internet café should not operate beyond midnight while its license will be revoked if any user surfs pornographic and "illegal" political websites. In early September 2002 Beijing issued a decree that banned the Internet search engines Google.com and AltaVista.com. More than 500,000 foreign websites have been blocked, despite Chinese official denial of blocking Google and other websites. On the eve of the opening of the 16th Party Congress, Liu Di, a 22-year-old-student, was arrested for her message posted in an Internet chatroom under the pseudonym "Stainless Steel Mouse".[10]

[8] *Ibid.*, pp. 107–111.

[9] See Shanthi Kalathil and Taylor C. Boas. 2003. *Open Networks, Closed Regimes: The Impact of the Internet on Authoritarian Rule*. Washington: The Carnegie Endowment for International Peace.

[10] Zhang Erping. "SARS: Unmasking censorship in China", *China Rights Forum*, No. 3, 2003, p. 47.

The use of these measures and mechanisms proves to be very effective for the authoritarian state to maintain its control over the mass media and information. They contradict Joseph Fewsmith's observation that "clearly, the transformation of communications technology, the growth of a contingent of dedicated Chinese journalists, the influence of reformers within the party, the presence of foreign reporters, and the impact of international pressure are making it increasingly difficult to control information".[11]

How did the Lack of Information Worsen the SARS Crisis

J. Mirsky points out: "Communist China's long obsession with secrecy is one cause of the present SARS (severe acute respiratory syndrome) crisis."[12] The first SARS case took place in Guangdong in November 16, 2002. "In the southern Chinese province of Guangdong (where SARS first appeared), the health department received a 'top secret' document from a government health committee on January 27 that contained disturbing information about a new pneumonia-like illness spreading in the region."[13] While Chinese leaders had access to top secret information about the outbreak of an epidemic, the general public knew little about it.

An internal warning was issued within the local government on February 7 in Guangdong. However, cell-phone and Internet messages spread the news about SARS between February 8 and 11. The first local press conference about SARS was held on February 11, 2003 in Guangzhou. However, all information and even the discussion on the Internet were suppressed in late February in Guangdong due to concerns about the local economy and stability. A free newspaper would have helped alert people of the existence of SARS, but the lack of the freedom of press made such an alternative impossible. Indeed, several SARS patients spread the disease to Hong Kong, Taiyuan, and Beijing without public awareness.

[11] Joseph Fewsmith. "China and the politics of SARS," *Current History*, Vol. 102, No. 665 (Sep. 2003), p. 254.
[12] Jonathan Mirsky. "How the Chinese spread SARS", *The New York Review*, Vol. L, No. 9 (9 May 2003), p. 42.
[13] *Ibid.*, p. 42.

If freedom of the press had been entrenched in the Chinese political system, then news about SARS in Guangdong in February 2003 would not have been easily suppressed by both the Chinese national and local governments. The outside world would have had an opportunity in the early stages of the outbreak to adopt preventative measures against SARS, and China would have also made the general public aware of the severity of the problem and contained SARS in the early stages. "More lives could have been saved had Beijing chosen not to cover up the issue for more than five months, and many more would certainly have died had the deception continued."[14]

Indeed, on February 18, 2003, Professor Zhong Nanshan, a doctor, urged the Guangdong government to release the information about the epidemic in an urgent meeting organized by the Department of Health. However, the local government adopted control measure. And when Professor Zhong proposed to develop a cooperation research project with Hong Kong University, he was regarded as the person who lacks "political caution".

It might be acceptable that the Beijing government did not act on SARS in February due to the uncertainty of the epidemic. It certainly was irresponsible of the Chinese government to withhold all information on SARS in March and early April, in particular when the governments in Hong Kong and Singapore took active measures against SARS and released information about SARS regularly. Beijing lost the entire month of March in its fight against SARS. From November 2002 to mid April 2003 Beijing responded to SARS with secrecy, denial, and cover-up. An epidemic could have been contained if Beijing had disclosed information.[15]

The cover-up was related to the transition of political power at the top. The new Party General Secretary Hu Jintao and his Politburo Standing Committee colleagues were to be approved and endorsed by the National Peoples' Congress in March 2003. "In order to ensure stability as the nation's two annual legislative assemblies got underway, hospital officials were forbidden to publicize what they had learned about SARS."[16] The Propaganda Department of the Party tends to suppress the bad news

[14] Zhang Erping. "SARS", p. 49.

[15] Arthur Waldron. "The Chinese sickness", *Commentary*, Vol. 116, No.1 (July–August 2003), p. 36.

[16] Jonathan Mirsky. "How the Chinese spread SARS", p. 42.

and disclose only the good news. Bad news makes the leaders look weak. Media officers and workers are instructed by the Propaganda Department of the Party on how a bad news should be presented or ignored.

In maintaining an authoritarian system of government, every politician must be a *knave*, and is proud to be and rewarded as a knave. It is a political maxim in an authoritarian system that every politician must be a knave. In North Korea, facts about the perpetual famine were denied. In Cuba, Fidel Castro told lies to his people every day. In China, lies, secrecy, denial and cover-up surrounded the SARS outbreak.[17] As J. Mirsky points out: "Any disaster, natural or man-made, can reflect badly on the Party, the government, officials, and of course all citizens. Low-ranking officials who cannot conceal secrets will not rise through the hierarchy, and the highest officials hesitate before telling some or all of the truth."[18]

Knavery, deception and lies are justified in the name of societal stability. A Shanghai doctor, an expert on epidemic diseases, expressed such a view: "You foreigners value each person's life more than we do because you have fewer people in your countries. Our primary concern is social stability, and if a few people's deaths are kept secret, it's worth it to keep things stable."[19] Indeed, to the Chinese authoritarian leaders, human life is little more than a statistic, and as long as the number of causalities remains within a permissible scope, they are an inevitable trade-off for maintaining social stability.[20]

Bureaucratic reports on the SARS figure to a higher authority often convey biased and distorted information. The actual SARS figure was under-reported for various purposes. On April 3, Zhang Wenkang, the Minister of Health, declared that Beijing only had 12 SARS cases and only three people had died. On April 4, Dr. Jiang Yanyong, a physician at Beijing's Chinese People's Liberation Army General Hospital (No. 301), blew the whistle on the actual number of SARS patients. He wrote a letter to the media and sent a fax to CCTV to reveal that there were

[17] Austin Bay. "How SARS scarred Asia's biggest tiger", *The Washington Time*, 20 May 2003, p.A20.

[18] Jonathan Mirsky. "How the Chinese spread SARS", p. 42.

[19] *Ibid.*, p. 42.

[20] Hu Ping. "SARS: The real story", *Beijing Spring*, Jun 2003.

Table 2. Summary of Probable SARS Cases with Onset of Illness from November 1, 2002 to July 31, 2003 (Revised September 26, 2003)

Areas	F	M	Total of cases	Median age (range)	Number of deaths	Case fatality ratio (%)	Number of imported case (%)	Number of HCW affected (%)	Date onset first probable case	Date onset last probable case
	Cumulative number of cases									
Canada	151	100	251	49(1–45)	43	17	5 (2)	109(43)	23-Feb-03	12-Jun-03
China (PRC)	2674	2607	5327	Pending	349	7	Not applicable	1002(19)	16-Nov-02	3-Jun-03
China, Hong Kong	977	778	1755	40(1–100)	299	17	Not applicable	386(22)	15-Feb-03	31-May-03
China, Macao	0	1	1	28	0	0	1(100)	0(0)	5-May-03	5-May-03
China, Taiwan	218	128	346	42(0–93)	37	11	21(6)	68(20)	25-Feb-03	15-Jun-03
Singapore	161	77	238	35(1–90)	33	14	8(3)	97(41)	25-Feb-03	5-May-03
Vietnam	39	24	63	43(20–76)	5	5	1(2)	36(57)	23-Feb-03	14-Apr-03

Source: http://www.who.int/csr/sars/country/table2003_09_23/en/, accessed on 18 Feb 2004.

60 SARS patients and seven had already died in a military Chinese media did not dare publish Dr. Jiang's letter. It was azine which finally released the true information as told b April 8, 2003.[21] While SARS patients in No. 301 military not under the Ministry of Health's purview due to the bifu itary-civilian authority, "the PLA's poor record in revealir to civilian authorities in the early days of the SARS ou attributed to the sense of autonomy and secrecy that has l ized the military in China".[22]

Originally, SARS was regarded as a local medical iss and March 2003. When it became a regional epidemic, it a political issue in April 2003. On April 7 Premier Wer China's Center for Disease Control and talked about the report on the SARS outbreak.[23] A special Politburo meeti April 17. On April 20, the Politburo Standing Committee the covering up of SARS cases and demanded the accur honest reporting of the SARS situation. Minister of Wenkang and Beijing Mayor Meng Xuenong were sacked National Task Force headed by Wu Yi was established. O the World Health Organization (WHO) lifted a travel issued against Beijing.

It should be stressed that the change in Chinese go tude was largely due to international pressure and globaliz ease. Wu Guoguang, a professor at the Chinese Universit commented: "In the past, lies did harm only to the Chir were killed as a result of lies did not know what actuall present, a single lie told by China will throw the whole w as if the world is faced with a formidable enemy."[24] The S spread to at least 28 countries including Australia, Brazil Africa, Spain, and the United States. The number o reached 8098 worldwide by July 31, 2003 (see Table 2).

[21] Susan Jakes. "Beijing's SARS attack: Doctor and party member ir more cases than officials will admit", *Time*, 8 Apr 2003.

[22] Joseph Fewsmith. "China and the politics of SARS", p. 253.

[23] *Ibid.*, p. 250.

[24] Wu Guoguang. "How to test the truth of speeches", *Hsin Pao*, Hong

points out: "Had this epidemic not plagued foreign countries and led to an international outrage, the Communist regime in Beijing would almost certainly have treated the epidemic with the same secrecy and indifference with which it has addressed the AIDS epidemic."[25] In order to maintain an image of being a good international citizen, Beijing cooperated with the WHO. Nevertheless, hospital staff members in Beijing told Pomfret of WHO that SARS patients were moved out when WHO officials were visiting.[26]

Closing a Window of Opportunity

From April–July 2003, the Propaganda Department of the Party maintained tight control over how the campaign against SARS was reported and clearly preferred the old ways. "The party was controlling information about the virus more closely than ever, and as for political change, SARS was not bringing it."[27] The official media had cast the party as the bulwark in the unfolding crisis.[28] The government criticized and warned against several journals and newspapers such as *Southern Weekend* that were very aggressive during the crisis. A propaganda official who suppressed media coverage of the outbreak in Guangdong was appointed editor of China's most liberal newspaper, *Southern Weekend.* This highlighted the party's determination to keep a tight grip on the press. The Propaganda Department still banned reports of Japanese sex-seeking tourists in Zhuhai after September 28, 2003 and on AIDS in Henan in October 2003.

Unwarranted descriptions and rumors contributed to the greater fear of SARS. Concealing and covering-up worsened the situation, and fuelled panic. It was necessary for a trusted authority to release factual information. Premier Wen Jiabao emphasized the need to build a reporting network running from provinces down to every village to provide

[25] Zhang Erping. "SARS", p. 49.

[26] Jonathan Mirsky. "How the Chinese spread SARS", p. 42.

[27] Arthur Waldron. "The Chinese sickness," p. 37.

[28] Pei Minxin. "Don't hold your breath for openness in China", *Financial Times*, 6 May 2003.

timely and objective information about SARS.[29] Gao Shiyi suggested that the government should collect facts, establish a crisis management team, release selected information, and frame the issue. He summarizes the strategies of the Chinese media in dealing with SARS: setting up a tone to inspire public emotion, reconstructing the image of the government as being capable of managing the crisis, and influencing public opinion so as to stabilize the society and maintain social order.[30]

Instead of learning a lesson and establishing an independent press system, the Chinese government stressed the art of controlling and managing information. It is the government that decides what sort of information and how and when it should be released to the public. The best way to defeat rumor is to release information. At the same time, the best way to reduce public fear is to conceal information. An art of governance is needed to achieve the balance between public accountability and control over information to reduce people's anxiety.

For the Chinese leadership, the old-styled campaign (*yundong*) proved successful in uniting the will of the masses, all religious organizations, and all democratic parties into a fortress.[31] A number of *People's Daily* commentary articles then appeared, strengthening the national spirit and even glorifying the virtue of the Chinese working class, building up to President Hu Jintao's call on May 1 to launch a "people's war" against SARS, calling for collective ethos, and relying on science and law.[32] In what Hu termed as the "people's war" against SARS, people were sure to be better informed, have a large say, and play a bigger role.[33]

China's traditional neighborhood committees and party cells in work units became the powerful weapon against SARS. Each committee had a list of every resident in every household in its area, making China one of the world's most highly organized societies. They also knew what each member of a household was doing, which school they attended, and

[29] *People's Daily*, 16 May 2003.

[30] http://www.cc.org.cn/wencui/030602200/0306022008.htm

[31] *People's Daily*, 30 Apr and 2 May 2003

[32] *People's Daily*, 30 Apr and 1, 12–15 May 2003.

[33] Xiong Lei. "SARS is making a change", *World Press Review*, Vol. 50, No. 7, Jul 2003.

where they worked. Through this network it was able to quickly detect sick people and keep them from infecting others.[34]

The SARS crisis created a small window of opportunity for the new leadership to open up the political system. However, this window was closed as soon as the SARS battle was over. In fact, the SARS crisis was a window of testing for Hu Jintao and Wen Jiabao's leadership. They passed the crucial test in this "homework". They removed Zheng Wenkang and Meng Xuenong decisively and visited SARS-hit communities. Hu Jintao even read his proposal on how to contain the epidemic on the Web. Ironically, as the Hu–Wen leadership established their authority through their handling of SARS, Western leaders respected them highly and did not pressure them on political reform, thus the incentive for them to carry out a substantial political reform program decreased.

What Lessons Should the Chinese Government Learn, According to Liberal Intellectuals

In the aftermath of the SARS crisis, Chinese intellectuals demanded more open reporting and accountability. Xu Jilin argues: "If a society faced with a crisis can only passively depend on government control, this in itself represents a latent crisis."[35] Putting people's interests first should be translated into a more liberal political system. A critical lesson from the SARS crisis is that people have the right to access information, the "right to know" (*zhiqingquan*). SARS linked the "right to know" with people's health. The victims, the families, and the public have the right to know the inside story. As Fewsmith argues: "By challenging the Chinese to consider not only the accountability of their government, but also issues of openness, trust, responsiveness, and the 'right to know', the SARS crisis seems likely to provide a major impetus to new thinking about relations between society and state."[36]

Zhang Shuguang, an economist, advocated that news control system be abolished and the freedom of press be promoted. He argued that SARS

[34] *South China Morning Post*, 16 May 2003.
[35] Joseph Fewsmith. "China and the politics of SARS", p. 254.
[36] *Ibid.*, p. 255.

revealed the fundamental deficiency of the existing system, that is, the lack of freedom of the press and the absence of freedom. If there were no control over the media, newspapers and journals could have reported the SARS outbreak, the diffusion of the SARS germs could have been prevented. In order to persuade the Chinese government to accept the freedom of the press, Zhang made a distinction between the freedom of speech and the freedom of decision-making. People have their freedom of speech to express whatever they want to say. However, this does not affect the government's right to make decisions. The Chinese government should not fear the consequence of the freedom of speech, and should be confident of its power and right to make decision and be responsible for the decision they make.[37] In contrast, Hu Ping, the former President of the Chinese Alliance for Democracy (CAD) in the U.S. from January 1988 to June 1991, defended his uncompromising position on the freedom of speech long time ago. Hu defined freedom of speech as the freedom to express different views, including wrong ones, which implies that expressing one's view may never lead to one being accused of a crime. This view goes against the official CCP definition, which states that freedom of speech is limited to what the leadership allows to be expressed.[38]

Wu Jinglian, an economist, urged the Chinese new leadership to seize the opportunity to promote political and social reforms, and to change China into an open, transparent and responsible government. He is worried that "the inertia of traditional thinking" might push China back onto "the old road".[39] "The old road" is the authoritarian way of controlling

[37] http://www.cc.org.cn/wencui/030602200/0306022000.htm.

[38] Hu also regards freedom of speech as the "fulcrum" upon which to rest a lever to "lift up this world", i.e., activate it into changing the totalitarian system. Hu is well aware of the problem that a totalitarian regime can only be overthrown if an autonomous oppositional force is established, and that the very aim of any totalitarian regime is exactly to prevent the rise of such a force. The only way out of this predicament, as Hu sees it, is to promote freedom of speech rather than to seek political power. He argues that freedom of speech strikes directly at one of the weakest spots in the totalitarian system: the power of modern totalitarianism is not only based on violent repression, but also on deception. See Hu Ping. 1988. *Gei wo yige zhidian (Give Me a Fulcrum)*. Taiwan: Lianjing chuban gongshi, pp. 14, 17–18, 48, 98.

[39] *The Economist*, 28 Jun 2003, p. 37.

information. Under an authoritarian system all information is regarded as "internal secrecy", ordinary people are denied the right to know, and governmental organizations and officials monopolize information for their power and interest. This system contributed to the diffusion of SARS around China. The fundamental solution to China's problems lies in the opening up and abolishing of traditional ways of controlling the media. Wu advocates strongly an alternative view of information. Information, except those related to public security and military affairs, is public resources, and should be free and equally accessible to people. In modern society, newspapers and journals, as well as radio and television stations, are powerful institutions for citizens to control government, rather than the "mouth of the Party's propaganda".[40] Chi Fulin, executive director of China Institute for Reform and Development, also argued: "The SARS crisis has proved that timely and objective publication of information is more important than anything. Any concealment or underreport will lead to unexpected consequences. The media need to have corresponding independence in publishing information in order to assume their social duties in a public crisis."[41]

Xu Wenli, a Chinese dissident who was imprisoned in 1998 for his involvement in the establishment of the Chinese Democratic Party in China and was released in 2002, said: "The SARS crisis in China shows that economic development alone is not enough to bring democracy to my country. When the epidemic of severe acute respiratory syndrome hit, the autocratic Chinese Communist Party concealed the origins and extent of the disease for months before it grudgingly gave in to international demands for transparency. And while SARS is a frightening phenomenon, a political system in such a condition that it would hide a dangerous disease from its own people and from the world is far more frightening."[42] Wang Dan, a former student leader in the 1989 Student

[40] Wu Jinglian. "SARS must create an open, transparent and responsible government in China", *Caijing* (Finance and Economics), No. 12, 2003.

[41] Chi Fulin. 2001. "Information system reform after SARS crisis", in Chi Fulin, ed., *Alarming Bell — China: SARS Crisis and System Reform*. Transition Report 2003, China Institute for Reform and Development. Beijing: Foreign Languages Press, pp. 138, 141.

[42] *Washington Post*, 19 May 2003, p. 19.

Demonstration in Tiananmen Square, asserted: "The epidemic will eventually pass. But it has shown that China's slowness and inappropriateness of response are unlikely to be remedied without political reform, particularly with regards to the mass media."[43]

WHY DIDN'T THE CHINESE GOVERNMENT LEARN A LESSON SUGGESTED BY LIBERAL INTELLECTUALS

Chinese liberal scholars think that the controlling and concealing of information by the Chinese government contributed to the outbreak of SARS. Chinese leaders however think otherwise. They are of the opinion that some of the more effective and successful measures against SARS are mobilization, "socialist spirit", the use of law, tough social control, and even the application of brute force.

China's political system proves to be resilient, cushioning the impact without substantial change in the area of the freedom of press. The success of the Party/State in the campaign against SARS indeed encourages it to draw different lessons. In a seminar on public health and economic development on June 17, 2003, Premier Wen Jiabao summarized the lessons that have been learnt from the SARS crisis: pay greater attention to and improve public health system; enhance the governmental capacity of handling an unexpected crisis; devote much more attention to the management of society; and attach importance to the coordination of economical and societal development. Wen hardly mentioned reform in the area of freedom of the press, except for "scientific and democratic" decision-making.[44]

Several factors contributed to this learning process. The severity and magnitude of SARS were not great, and the duration of SARS was short, so SARS only had a marginal impact on economic development and political reform. If the actual damage of SARS were serious, its shocking effects were even greater. Moreover, the campaign against SARS relied on the government's resources and mobilization. The isolation practice required a tough control and justified a severe restriction on personal

[43] Wang Dan. "Epidemic shows China's weaknesses", *Taipei Times*, 4 May 2003.
[44] *Lookout News Weekly*, No. 25, 23 Jun 2003, p. 6.

liberty. A call for personal liberty cannot cure the SARS patient. Too much civic liberty escalated the problem in Taiwan with SARS patients running out of hospital, local leaders in Xingzhu county refusing to accept SARS patient transferred from Taipei, and citizens disobeying quarantine order.

A note of caution is also needed. In the democratic state of Canada where the freedom of press is well protected, it was not spared from a SARS outbreak. On the other hand, the undemocratic administration in Hong Kong and the authoritarian government in Singapore disclosed rather than concealed SARS information in March 2003. Indeed, according to WHO, Hong Kong has been exemplary in its reporting and transparency even when the economic consequences of doing so were known to be significant.

Here it is important to note that information control by the Chinese authoritarian state during the early stages worsened the situation. The authoritarian regime of China was a facilitating factor that helped to speed up the spread of SARS. However, the authoritarian government of Singapore disclosed information to the general public in order to contain the outbreak of SARS. Of a more important note is that in curing SARS, different political regimes did very little as it is considered purely a medical problem. Liberals should not be blind to the fact that SARS is a natural disease, and fighting against it requires isolation and tough control.

Undoubtedly while the Chinese authoritarian government is capable of controlling information due to the lack of the freedom of press, it is vice versa for the democratic government. All governments tend to control information about the uncertainty of an epidemic. The difference lies in the existence of independent press and media and various institutional alternatives such as non-governmental organizations to governmental source in democratic states. Above all, people in a democratic regime have the right to access information, and a democratic government is under pressure to share information with its people.

Conclusion

If China wants to be a it must improve on the quality of its governance and institutionalize an honest regime in which the freedom of the press is a necessary component. How does the Chinese government win the trust of the international community? Wu Guoguang once suggested: "If Hu Jintao and Wen Jiabao want to enjoy the trust of the people and if the Chinese government wants to enjoy the trust of the world, they should immediately change the way they are treating Dr. Jiang. If Hu or Wen says openly, 'Dr. Jiang Yanyong is a responsible good citizen and we would like to thank him on behalf of the people,' the trustworthiness of any statement made by the Chinese government would immediately increase by a big margin."[45] Contrary to Wu's suggestion, Dr. Jiang Yanyong was not only forbidden to meet foreign journalists, he was also criticized in a circular issued by the PLA. Angered by this, Professor Wu Jinglian hailed Dr. Jiang as the hero who made a great contribution to China and the Chinese people. In reply, Dr. Jiang said that he is only an honest doctor, nothing more. It is ordinary Chinese folks like Dr. Jiang, whose honesty spells hope for China's future.

In the case of SARS, the Chinese authoritarian system proves to be resilient, adaptive and responsive. Though the natural SARS epidemic is temporarily over, the political "SARS" ("scandal authoritarian regime syndrome") remains. Lies, secrecy, and knavery are still a daily practice. The authoritarian regime still exercises its control over information through sophisticated mechanisms as illustrated in Section 1, and it becomes more cunning and skillful in controlling and disclosing information. The freedom of the press is a long way from becoming a reality. Chinese scientists lost their battle to be the first to discover the secret of the SARS germs;[46] Chinese liberals lost their fight to push Chinese political reform further; the lives of 349 dead patients, and 5,329 affected patients seem to be wasted. A genuine lesson has yet to be learned.

[45] Wu Guoguang. "How to test the truth of speeches".

[46] See Cao Cong. "Chinese scientists were defeated by SARS", a chapter included in this volume.

Chapter 8

The Hong Kong SAR Government, Civil Society and SARS

ELSPETH THOMSON AND YOW CHEUN HOE

INTRODUCTION

By February 10 2003, public fear was intensifying in Hong Kong following newspaper reports as well as text messages on mobile phones and the Internet, of an unusual, fatal pneumonia-like epidemic in the adjacent Chinese province of Guangdong where there was panic-buying of antibiotics, masks, white vinegar, and herbal medicines believed to enhance immunity.[1] Receiving no confirmation from the Special Administration Region (SAR) government, Hong Kong citizens also scrambled to buy these. The actual entry of severe acute respiratory syndrome (SARS) into Hong Kong occurred on February 21 when a Guangzhou kidney specialist, Professor Liu Jianlun, checked into the Metropole Hotel and stayed for one night. From there, SARS began to spread around the world when he unknowingly infected other hotel guests who travelled from Hong Kong to Vietnam, Singapore, and Canada. Professor Liu was admitted to the Kwong Wah Hospital on February 22 and succumbed on March 4.[2] Not until March 12 did the Department of Health announce the outbreak of SARS in the Prince of Wales Hospital.[3] On March 27, more

[1] "It all started at the Metropole", *Straits Times*, 22 Jul 2003. In Chinese society, white vinegar is typically used as an all-purpose disinfectant.

[2] SARS Expert Committee. *SARS Expert Committee Report*, Hong Kong, 2 Oct 2003, at http://www.sars-expertcom.gov.hk, pp. 18–21, 198.

[3] *Ibid.*, p. 23.

than two weeks after the crisis began, Hong Kong Chief Executive Tung Chee-hwa addressed the public for the first time on SARS to announce quarantine and screening programs.[4]

The onset of SARS in Hong Kong could hardly have come at a worse time. Though the people of Hong Kong were hopeful when the British government handed over the Territory to Mainland China on July 1, 1997 that all would be well, right from the start the new administration was perceived as fundamentally dysfunctional. When the first case of SARS entered the Territory and began to spread quickly, there were already several political issues upsetting the general population. This new problem immediately added to the maelstrom and successfully united critical public opposition. As in the other cities where it hit, the authorities and public alike did not know exactly what it was that struck them, and therefore how to deal with it.

The first several sections of this paper briefly outline the Hong Kong government's response to the crisis, i.e., the measures taken to try to contain the virus and reduce its impact socially and economically, and some of the problems with these. This is followed by an analysis of the political backdrop before and after the outbreak of the virus, and the significance of the crisis in terms of civil society.

Managing the Crisis

Government Response

Travel advisories

On April 2, the World Health Organization (WHO) issued a travel advisory recommending that persons travelling to Hong Kong and Guangdong Province consider postponing all but essential travel.[5] It was the strictest travel advisory in its 55-year history. The U.S. State Department imposed a travel warning on April 16 and allowed its nonessential staff to leave the Territory.

[4] "Hong Kong's SARS whitewash", *Asian Wall Street Journal*, 7 Oct 2003, p. A 11.

[5] See World Health Organization (WHO) website: http://www.who.int/csr/sarsarchive/2003_04_02/en/, Oct 2003.

The WHO travel advisory was lifted on May 23, and on June 2, Hong Kong officials launched a massive campaign across the Untied Kingdom to persuade business and leisure travellers that the city was safe. On June 11, the U.S. State Department ended its travel warning and authorized the return of American government employees.

Hong Kong was finally removed from the WHO's list of SARS infected areas on June 23 after 20 days had passed without any fresh outbreaks in the Territory.

Screening procedures at immigration control points

On March 29, all of the Territory's immigration control checkpoints adopted health-declaration procedures. The Department of Health stationed officers at each checkpoint to check if anyone coming into Hong Kong showed signs of atypical pneumonia. Starting from April 17, passengers leaving the Territory by plane had their temperatures taken before they checked in for their flights. If they were found to have a fever, they would be asked to see a doctor at the airport — at their own expense — who would determine the possibility of their suffering from SARS.

Following a report in a local paper that as many as 5,000 air travellers a day managed to escape having their temperature taken, on April 25, health officers at Hong Kong's Chek Lap Kok Airport began to check the temperatures of all incoming passengers as well as those in transit, not just outgoing passengers.

School closures

Only after many parents decided to keep their children at home — potentially an offence under the Education Ordinance — were schools closed. The date chosen to close the schools, March 27, was the same date as in Singapore. It was initially announced that kindergartens, primary and secondary schools, special schools and day courses would be closed from this date to April 21, and the universities to April 13. Later the Hong Kong Education and Manpower Bureau decided that students of secondary level three and above would return to their schools on April 22, junior secondary students would return on the 28th, and primary and special school students would return in stages from early to mid May.[6]

Quarantine measures

The Department of Health invoked the Quarantine and Prevention of Disease Ordinance on March 31. At the same time, Secretary for Health, Welfare and Food, Dr. Yeoh Eng-Keong, announced the isolation of Block E of Amoy Gardens, a densely-populated housing estate situated in the district of Ngau Tau Kok, after 213 residents there, half of which lived in that particular block, came down with the virus.[7] A day later, 241 residents put in isolation there were moved to government holiday villages. This isolation order ended on April 9 at midnight. Initially it was conjectured that this outbreak was being spread through the drainage and sewage system or by cockroaches, but was traced to a man from Shenzhen who regularly received haemodialysis at the Prince of Wales Hospital.[8] When in Hong Kong, he stayed at his brother's flat in Amoy Gardens (more details below).

On April 10, the government announced that it would strictly enforce home quarantine for people known to have had close contact with someone who had the disease, including all members of the patient's household. Starting from April 14, anyone under home quarantine having had close contact with someone confirmed to have the virus was prevented from leaving Hong Kong. On April 24, Director of Health Dr. Margaret Chan Fung-Fu announced that beginning from the next day, home-confinement arrangements for families of atypical pneumonia patients would extend to "suspect" cases.

Healthcare system and lab work

Responding to media reports, on April 1, Dr. Margaret Chan refuted rumours that Hong Kong would declare itself an infected area. However,

[6] See Hong Kong government press releases: http://www.emb.gov.hk/emb/eng/info/press/2003/list_200303.html; http://www.emb.gov.hk/emb/eng/info/press/2003/ list_200304.html; http://www.emb.gov.hk/emb/eng/info/press/2003/list_200305.html, Oct 2003.

[7] Eventually, 329 residents of Amoy Gardens became infected and 42 died. *SARS Expert Committee Report*, p. 40.

[8] *SARS Expert Committee Report*, pp. 44, 52.

WHO experts arrived in Hong Kong on the 27th and joined the Department of Health's ongoing investigation into environmental factors that were possibly aiding the spread of the virus.

On May 6, WHO's Executive Director for Disease, Dr. David Heymann held a videoconference with Hong Kong officials to discuss WHO's travel advisory, and on the 28th, Tung announced plans for a three-month review of the city's health system by a panel of international medical experts. The 11-member body, consisting of experts from the United States, Britain, Australia, Hong Kong, and Mainland China were to examine the Territory's health facilities to better prepare for future viral outbreaks.

Researchers at Hong Kong universities, in collaboration with scientists at Guangzhou Medical College and Fudan University in Shanghai in late May completed the first stage of developing vaccines. The next step was to test it in animals, firstly for safety, and secondly to discover whether it produced a protective immune response.

On June 6, Hong Kong researchers said they had found the virus in civet cats in Guangdong Province, and that they believed it jumped from these animals to humans.[9] As a precaution, the Hong Kong government announced on June 9 it would temporarily ban the import of civet meat, and officials warned people to stay away from the few civet cats found in the wild.

On June 23, when WHO removed Hong Kong from its list of SARS-affected areas, Beijing, Toronto, and Taiwan remained on the list. Health Secretary Yeoh chose that day to announce plans to build 1,000 isolation rooms to prevent a repeat of hundreds of hospital patients becoming infected.

Measures to revive the economy

Since late 1997, Hong Kong's economy had been in decline. The SARS outbreak worsened an already bleak situation. In all, over the four months through July, Hong Kong's budget deficit widened by 11%, an increase the government attributed to the lower consumer spending and

[9] Civet cat meat is eaten as a delicacy in southern China. These nocturnal animals which are related to the mongoose and resemble raccoons or weasels, are also raised for their fur and musk.

tourism revenues due to SARS, as well as the extra spending allocated towards measures aimed at containing SARS.[10] The deficit from April to July widened to HK$44.7 billion (US$5.7 billion) compared to HK$40.1 billion over the same period in 2002. Revenue fell 9.6% to HK$34.9 billion and spending increased 1.1% to HK$79.6 billion.

In an attempt to relieve the worst-hit sectors, Tung outlined a package of economic-relief measures on April 23 worth about HK$11.8 billion. On May 19, more than 1,000 retailers and restaurants joined forces to launch "Come Back Hong Kong" to woo customers back into shops. Members who signed up were given discounts at shops and other incentives to spend. The declaration by WHO that the Territory was SARS-free, was marked by the launching of a HK$400 million campaign planned to extend over nine months. Large discounts were announced to lure back foreign visitors in particular.

PROBLEMS WITH THE GOVERNMENT'S RESPONSE

The Hong Kong government's success in handling the SARS outbreak can be measured in terms of: (1) the number of people afflicted by the disease and the speed at which its spread was halted; and (2) governmental mistakes and incohesive action.

Number of People Afflicted by the Disease and Speed in Halting its Spread

The epidemic began in Hong Kong on March 10 when 11 healthcare workers from ward 8A of the Prince of Wales Hospital simultaneously reported themselves too ill to report for their shifts. The first death occurred on March 17. Over 100 people were dead by April 23, and over 200 by May 7. By June 28, the day of the final death as of time-of-writing, the toll was just short of 300 at 298 (see Figures 1 and 2). Deaths per day peaked at 13 on April 27, and the death of the first of three healthcare workers occurred on May 22.

[10] Cathy Chan. "SARS helps widen Hong Kong deficit", *International Herald Tribune*, 1 Sept 2003.

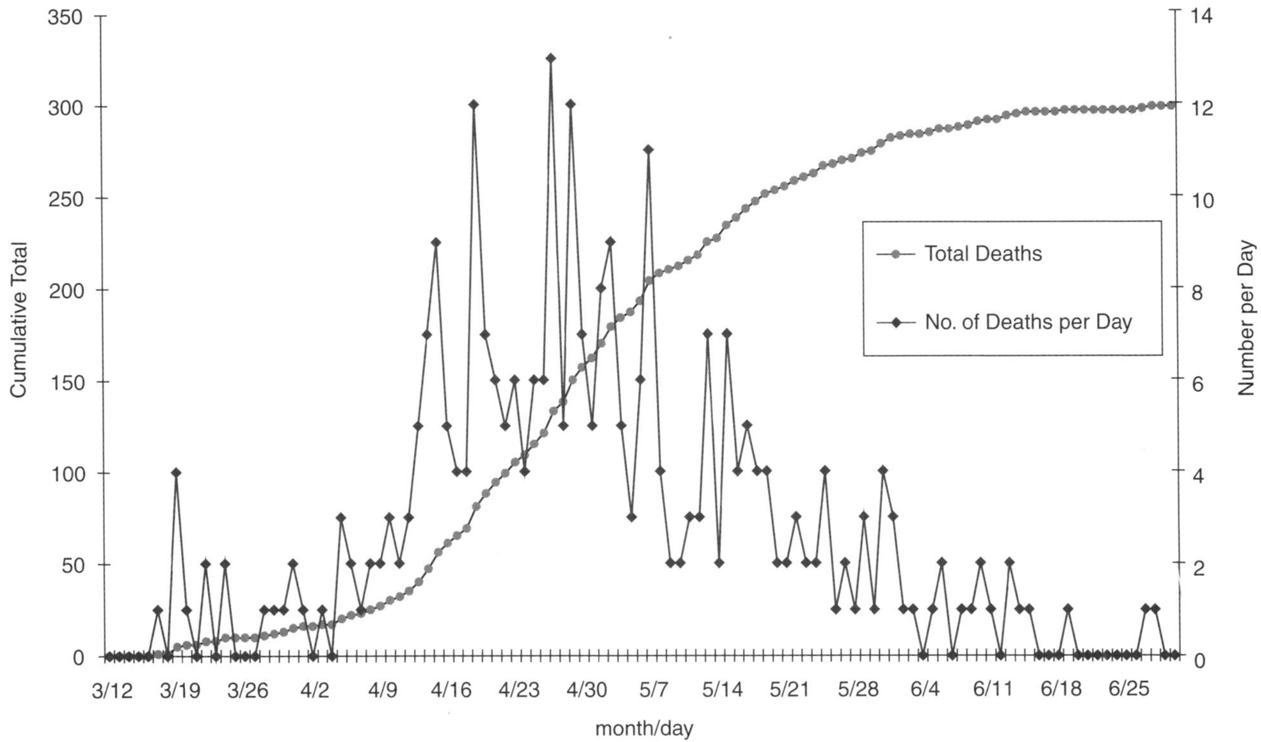

Figure 1. Deaths from SARS in Hong Kong as of June 2003

Source: "SARS updated charts and figures in Hong Kong", Hong Kong University of Science & Technology, at http://ihome.ust.hk/~bo_cckae/kivin/sars.html.

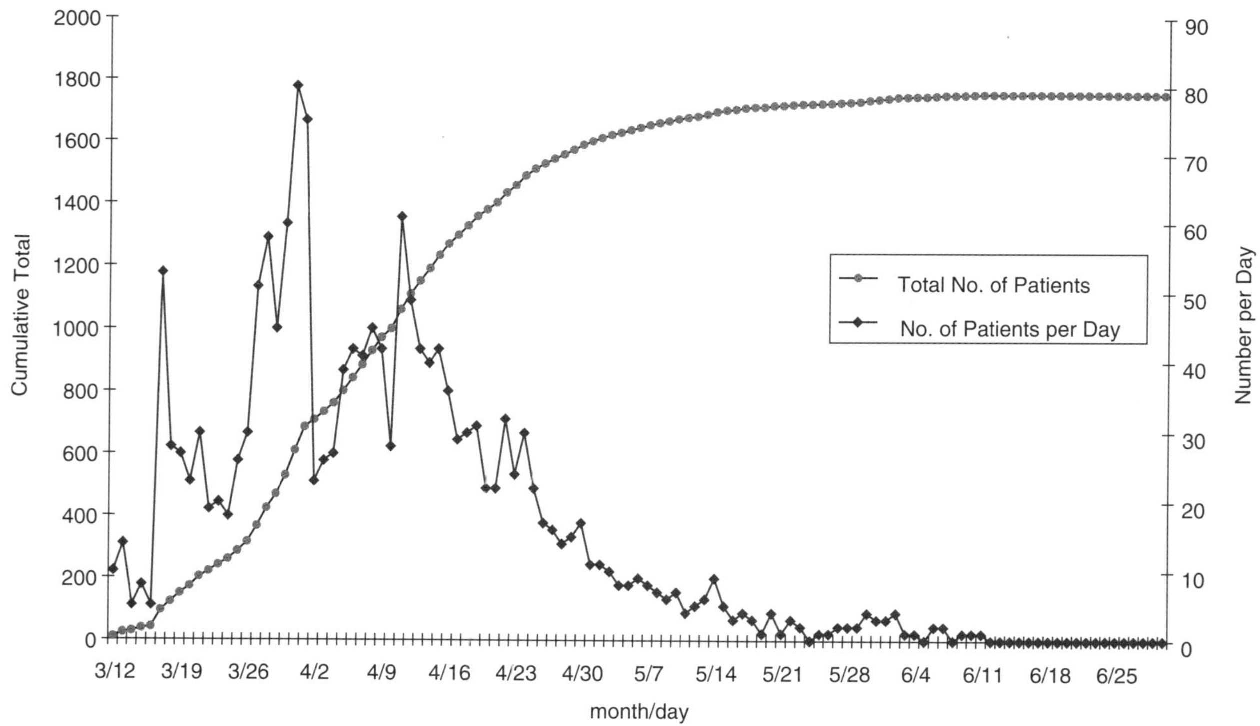

Figure 2. Officially Confirmed SARS Patients in Hong Kong as of June 2003

Source: "SARS updated charts and figures in Hong Kong", Hong Kong University of Science & Technology, at http://ihome.ust.hk/~bo_cckae/kivin/sars.html.

The spread of the disease was most rapid from about April 12 to May 14. Total confirmed cases increased from 0 to 100 between March 12 and 18. Only three days later, there were over 200. By the end of the month there were over 600, and by mid-April, over 1,200. Over the month of May, the rate slowed considerably, increasing from 1,600 to 1,739, a total of about 140 cases. The first day without any new cases was May 24, and after June 11 there were no new cases reported. The total since then has remained at 1,755. Globally, Hong Kong was the second most severely hit, after Mainland China which had 5,327 cases and 349 deaths.[11] For comparison, there were 665 cases and 180 deaths on Taiwan, 251 cases and 41 deaths in Canada, 238 cases and 33 deaths in Singapore, and 63 cases and 5 deaths in Vietnam.

The virus reached every corner of the Territory. At its peak, on April 14, as many as 176 buildings were identified with confirmed SARS cases (see Figure 3). Each of these cases was hospitalized for treatment.[12] The worst affected areas were the districts of Kwun Tong in Kowloon, and Shatin and Taipo in the New Territories. From June 8 on, the final new cases all came from the Eastern New Territories.

It was 106 days between the onset date of the first probable case in Hong Kong and the last (from February 15 to May 31).[13] The corresponding durations were 222 days in China (November 16 to June 25), 111 days in Taiwan (February 25 to June 15), 110 days in Canada (February 23 to June 12), 70 days in Singapore (February 25 to May 5), and 51 days in Vietnam (February 23 to April 14).

According to Hong Kong Public Doctors' Association president Leung Ka Lau, of the four cities which acquired the virus almost simultaneously when the doctor from Guangdong stayed at the Metropole Hotel on February 21: "Hong Kong suffered from an unacceptably large-scale outbreak, resulting in more than 200 additional and avoidable deaths."

[11] *SARS Expert Committee Report*, p. 5.

[12] Two lists of buildings were compiled from information provided by patients with confirmed/suspected diagnosis of SARS. If there were no further cases in ten days or the suspected patient was later found not to be suffering from SARS, the names of the buildings were taken off the relevant list. See http://www.info.gov.HongKong/dh/diseases/ap/eng/bldgindex.htm, Oct 2003.

[13] Calculated from *SARS Expert Committee Report*, p. 79.

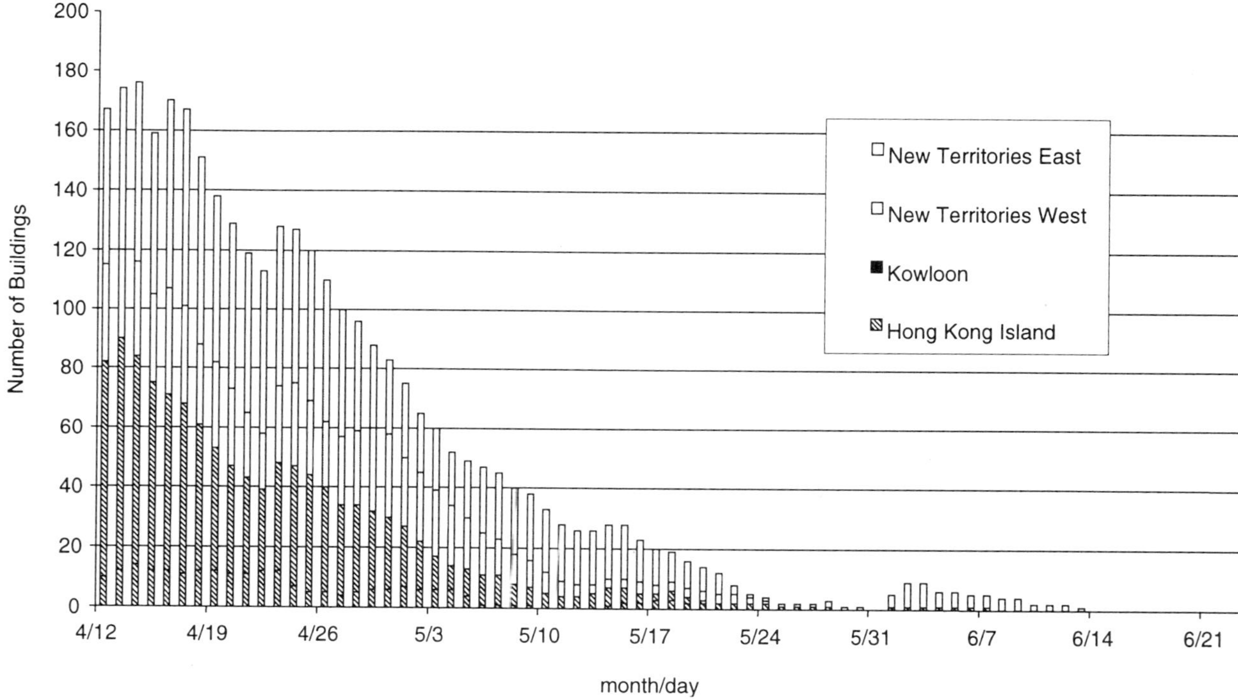

Figure 3. Number of Buildings with Confirmed SARS Patients by Region and Date of Posting onto the Hong Kong Department of Health Website as of June 2003

Source: Hong Kong Department of Health, at http://www.info.gov.hk/dh/diseases/ap/eng/bldgcht.htm. Information was first posted at this site on 12 Apr 2003.

He maintained: "From a scientific and professional point of view, the four cities were in a similar position when the epidemics started."[14]

The infection and death rates in Hong Kong were indeed high. However, the government and people of Hong Kong managed to contain it faster than did Canada and Taiwan. Of the total cases, 17.1% died in Hong Kong, 27.1% in Taiwan, 16.3% in Canada, 13.9% in Singapore, 7.9% in Vietnam, and 6.6% in China.[15]

Mistakes and Incohesion

Mistake no. 1 — Delayed, mixed messages. By March 12, ten people were infected with SARS, but it was only a fortnight later, on March 27, that Dr Yeoh, admitted that Hong Kong had indeed been hit by SARS and it was necessary to implement certain measures.[16] Initially the government was over-reassuring and did not inform the public of the actual gravity of the situation.[17] Public sector workers claimed they were unnecessarily exposed to danger. On the one hand, the government advised medical people to take no chances, but at the same time was telling the world there was nothing to worry about. A government doctor is quoted as saying: "Had the public been properly warned of the severity of the virus and the possibility that it had spread within the community, the number of non-medical patients might not have grown that fast."[18]

The Hong Kong government delayed closing the schools because the Secretary of Education Arthur Li and the Secretary of Health, Dr. Yeoh,

[14] In a letter entitled "A tale of four cities" written by K. L. Leung, President of the Hong Kong Public Doctors' Association, sent by fax and post on June 3, 2003 to Tung Chee Hwa, at http://137.189.140.4/pda/sars/attachment/ID116_LetterToTung030603.doc, Oct 2003.

[15] *SARS Expert Committee Report*, pp. 78–80.

[16] Wong Kwok Wah and Janus Lam. "HK plays down pneumonia fears", *Asia Times Online*, 18 Mar 2003 (31 May 2003).

[17] Phar Kim Beng. "SARS threatens countries' political health", *Asia Times Online*, 9 Apr 2003 (31 May 2003).

[18] Wong Kwok Wah and Atol staff reporters. "Paranoia prevails in SARS' ground zero", *Asia Times Online*, 28 Mar 2003 (1 Jun 2003).

argued that this step would be harmful to the Territory's economy. Apropos this, one doctor remarked: "It can only be assumed that bureaucratic considerations had taken precedence over professional judgements."[19] By contrast, the information and directives given by Singapore and Vietnamese governments over the same period, i.e., when little was known about the disease anywhere, were much less ambiguous. These governments were less concerned with minimizing economic damage.

Mistake no. 2 — Permitting a diagnosed case of atypical pneumonia treated at the Prince of Wales Hospital to return home. The "index patient" from the Amoy Gardens, actually a resident of Shenzhen, was a regular kidney patient at the hospital and had arrived unwell at the hospital on the 15th for his dialysis.[20] With a high fever and diarrhea, he was promptly diagnosed as a suspected case of atypical pneumonia, and given antibiotics and anti-flu treatment. By the 19th, he was much improved and the chest x-ray indicated almost complete resolution of the changes caused by the pneumonia. Lab tests showed he had had influenza type A. Ideally, the doctors would have kept this patient in quarantine. However, he was discharged and spent the night at his brother's home in Amoy Gardens, then returned to Shenzhen on the 20th, then back to the Prince of Wales Hospital on the 22nd for dialysis. At that point, he required urgent treatment for pneumonia and was admitted into the intensive care unit the following day.

Mistake no. 3 — Delays in quarantine procedures generally. Initially, people in close contact with infected people — household members and other close contacts — were not immediately quarantined, but ordered to visit special clinics for daily checkups, i.e., they were potentially spreading the disease rapidly! They were advised not to go to work or school for at least seven days and granted formal sick leave. The Department of Health kept in contact with them over the phone. On March 31, the "household contacts" were required to report for daily inspection at a designated medical center for ten days. They were asked not to venture outside apart from these daily trips for medical surveillance. It was not until

[19] *Ibid.*

[20] *SARS Expert Committee Report*, pp. 40–53. This patient fully recovered and was ultimately discharged June 2.

April 4 that these people were ordered to quarantine themselves at home for ten days. No visitors were permitted other than public health nurses who regularly checked them and the police who made spot checks so as to ensure compliance.

The "other close contacts" were not ordered to remain in their homes until April 25. Throughout this time they continued their daily trips to the medical centers dispersed around the Territory. Sometimes there were long queues at these centers, and a request by the Amoy Gardens Owners' Committee to set up a medical examination post right on the estate, was turned down.

Mistake no. 4 — Delayed announcement at Hong Kong Baptist Hospital. This privately-run hospital was reprimanded for failing to notify the authorities of the outbreak of SARS on its premises. Dr. Margaret Chan accused the head of the facility of failing to notify promptly the authorities as well as patients and their families of an outbreak of SARS in April.[21] She said the Hospital "failed to take patient's rights seriously" by failing to comply with the department's instructions, issued on March 19 to report all suspected SARS cases to officials. A total of 13 patients and medical workers were infected at the hospital, and one patient died. Action was taken swiftly — the head of the hospital, Dr. Tsang Chin Wah, was fired effective from May 26.

Public Response

Disaffected Already

Long before the SARS outbreak, many Hong Kongers were expressing great disappointment with their government which is executive-style, not popularly elected. Currently, only 24 members of the 60-seat Legislative Council are directly elected, and of the remaining seats, 30 are elected from professional or occupational constituencies and six by an 800-strong pro-Beijing Committee. Thus, with the support of lawmakers from the pro-business Liberal Party and the pro-Beijing Democratic

[21] Patsy Moy. "Hospital is scolded for keeping SARS cases quiet", *South China Morning Post*, 3 Jun 2003.

Alliance for the Betterment of Hong Kong, Tung has had little difficulty finding the numbers to pass government laws. Immediately following the Handover, much of the populace began to feel it had little ability to influence the destiny of the Territory, and became frustrated by the fact that most of the people in the top positions had little political experience.

The Asian financial crisis which began soon after the British Government left in 1997, had devastating effects on Hong Kong especially. The city had always prided itself on virtually no unemployment, and it suddenly found itself with a rate above 8%. In the following year, a frightening outbreak of avian flu occurred, and there were numerous questionable pronouncements pertaining to right of abode. The repeated appointment of international advisory panels, composed of "experts" who generally knew very little about local conditions, to solve various problems in the Territory raised the growing level of cynicism. In April 2002, Tung introduced a Principal Officials Accountability System, but the general consensus among the public was that it was brought in too hastily. Ironically, its credibility was severely damaged by the "penny stocks fiasco" which began July 2002.[22]

Instead of dealing with the various problems swiftly and directly, Tung prolonged the irritation by postponing the announcement of his Policy Address for three months, in order to buy time for all parties to get "on track". Then the public became enraged upon learning that the Financial Secretary conveniently timed the purchase of a family car just before announcing in his Budget Speech the introduction of higher taxes on luxury cars.

In the months immediately prior to the outbreak of SARS, the Tung administration seemed almost entirely fixated on passing Article 23 of the Basic Law (the SAR's mini-constitution), which was to make illegal any act of treason, secession, sedition, subversion against the Central People's Government, or theft of state secrets, and prohibited political

[22] The penny stocks fiasco was sparked when a consultation paper issued by the Hong Kong Exchange proposed the de-listing of certain penny stocks that had failed to meet certain criteria such as market cap, shareholders equity, profitability, clean audit reports and nominal share prices. This resulted in a crash of micro-cap stocks on a Friday, and a frantic withdrawal of the proposals on the Sunday.

organizations or bodies of the region from establishing ties with foreign political organizations or bodies. As the economy, in terms of unemployment, pay cuts, and real estate prices which had declined by two-thirds since 1997, had never been worse, and government economists themselves were saying that the process of economic re-structuring could take a long time, the people were continuously hoping for specific measures aimed at cushioning the difficulties. The persistence in pushing through legislation which at this time especially, seemed unnecessary, soured the public's view of its leadership yet further.

Making matters worse, the government continued to boast the benefits of its small size and low and simple tax regime. It prided itself on being one of the most laissez-faire economies in the world. There had always been virtually nothing offered in terms of unemployment insurance or other social safety nets. At the same time, the government openly propped up the property market, and helped wealthy, albeit over-extended, big developers.

Once the public understood that a highly contagious disease had struck Hong Kong, the fear of infection caused people to minimize their exposure by staying away from crowded places. They did not shop, go to banks, restaurants, etc. Air traffic to the Territory virtually ceased and hotels were empty for weeks. Salaries in all non-governmental sectors were affected and the Hong Kong economy already in serious trouble, sunk further.

Many Hong Kongers seemed to make a fairly clear distinction between, on the one hand, the mistakes on the medical side, i.e., the initially major shortcomings in the infection control facilities and procedures within almost all the hospitals and clinics, and on the other, the unclear information and directives issued by the government and poor communications among the departments involved. Far less forgiving of the latter, they immediately accused the government of a slow and clumsy response and believed that Tung was once again not being sufficiently responsive to public concerns and not holding his staff accountable. They were angry with the bureaucrats and, perhaps unfairly, compared them to those in Singapore.

Beginning June 30, the Chinese Premier, Wen Jiabao, spent three days in the Territory. Besides bringing the Closer Economic Partnership Agreement (CEPA), a free-trade agreement with the Mainland designed to bring the two economies even closer, he also attended a ceremony commending Hong Kong's heroes in the medical profession and others involved. At Amoy Gardens, he offered comfort to the victim's families. Significantly, on the following day, a Hong Kong newspaper described him as "a man of the people; liberal-minded; a bearer of kind words".

Almost as soon as he left, on the sixth anniversary of the Handover on July 1, a demonstration was held. The numbers which gathered — officially half a million, but possibly up to 700,000, and far higher than in previous years — shocked both the Hong Kong and Chinese governments.[23] Other rallies were also held on July 9 (about 50,000 people) and July 13 (about 15,000). All of these were largely geared to forcing the government to withdraw Article 23, but were also an expression of anger at the rising unemployment, small business bankruptcies, home-mortgage foreclosures, home ownership with negative equity, potentially higher taxes, reforms to education and public health, and crime.[24]

The make-up of the protests was worrying — most of the demonstrators were middle class and well-educated, many of them traditional Liberal Party supporters. Very significantly, there was no violence or thuggery accompanying the protest. All commercial outlets remained open and there were no arrests. In the end, the protests did have the desired effect. They forced the government to soften, then postpone the anti-subversion bill.

SIGNIFICANCE OF THE CRISIS

SARS was an external shock that was completely unpredicted. Not surprisingly, the eventual emergency response of the government was as in a war, i.e., the government measures were inherently undemocratic, and there were bound to be mistakes. SARS caused cracks to appear in the functioning of all the healthcare delivery systems and administrations around the world that suddenly had to cope with it. It is fair to say that

[23] Opinion surveys suggest that 16% of the population participated in the demonstration, putting the number at well over 600,000. See Frank Ching. "Against the tide", *South China Morning Post*, 23 Oct 2003, p. A 12.

[24] Henry C. K. Liu. "Why Hong Kong is in crisis", *Asia Times Online*, 4 Jul 2003 (4 Jul 2003).

in all the countries that were hit, fighting among various levels of government affected front-line healthcare workers, and that announcements and instructions to the public about the magnitude of the crisis were inconsistent and unclear.

In the initial stages, none of the health professionals in Hong Kong knew what they were dealing with. Moreover, according to recent statistics, there had been up to 1,400 cases of pneumonia admitted into Hong Kong hospitals per month.[25] There had also, for some time, been various strains of avian flu appearing in the region. It took some weeks before the international medical authorities reached agreement on what were the classic symptoms and means of transmission. It was difficult for any government to offer clear instructions.

Although there was no doubt that several mistakes were made, overall, Hong Kong's medical authorities' handling of SARS, though not nearly as effective as in Singapore, was much better than China's, Taiwan's or Canada's.

WTO's Executive Director of Communicable Diseases, Dr. David Heymann, was full of praise for the way Hong Kong handled the crisis, saying: "Had Hong Kong not been as transparent as it had been, the world would be much behind in understanding this outbreak. It's the data collected in Hong Kong and also Singapore which has been used by scientists throughout the world to understand so much about this outbreak".[26] Referring to contact tracing done by the Department of Health and police through the SARS and Major Incident Investigation and Disaster Support Program, he remarked: "It's a very unique way of tracing contacts. It will likely be copied in the future and imitated throughout the world. It's a very important marriage of databases." He also lauded Hong Kong scientists for their contribution to the knowledge base of SARS — work on finding the cause, on diagnostic tests and animal studies done in collaboration with mainland researchers.

Another doctor from WTO, Dr. Mike Ryan, was extremely impressed by the way in which Hong Kong had managed the epidemic, saying: "In

[25] *SARS Expert Committee Report*, p. 68.

[26] Hong Kong government press release, http://www.info.gov.hk/gia/general/brandhk/0616224.htm, Oct 2003.

fact, it is a model for the world. The leadership shown by Dr. Yeoh and the teams in the public health sector has been exemplary."[27]

The Dean of Medicine at University of Toronto, Dr. David Naylor said: "Hong Kong officials were able to fill medical journals with first-class studies while managing a much bigger outbreak." By contrast, "we [medical authorities in Canada] were arguing over who owned the data".[28]

This is not to say that the system worked flawlessly. One major adjustment called for in the wake of the crisis was creation of a single Secretary for Public Health position. When the crisis hit, Yeoh Eng-Keong was Secretary for Health, Welfare and Food. Many doctors, such as Dr. Lee Shiu-Hung, former Director of Health, and now Professor of Community Medicine at Chinese University, recommended that it was too large a portfolio for one person to manage well, accounting for more than 30% of the entire budget.[29] He also gave the opinion that the government had focused too much on hospital services and too little on public health.

Dr. Lee further noted that the Department of Health, which is responsible for health prevention and controlling infectious disease, was operating on a budget just a tenth that of the Hospital Authority. "We need a full-time person to take up public health. The existing role of the director of health is on the executive level. The director just implements the policies set by the secretary." He also argued that "Hong Kong should have its own center for disease control and prevention, with support from experts in microbiology, epidemiology and community medicine".

Another recommendation, by Lo Wing-Lok, the legislator representing the medical profession, was that "the director of health should be given more power. [He] should report directly to the chief executive so he or she can make medical decisions to protect lives [which] would not be affected by political or economic considerations".[30]

[27] "Hong Kong praised for its handing of SARS", at http://www.info.gov.hk, 14 Jun 2003.
[28] "Government bungled handling of SARS: Doctor", *CBCnews Online*, 17 Sept 2003 (18 Sept 2003).
[29] Ella Lee. "Call for a ministry dedicated to promoting public health", *South China Morning Post*, 4 Jun 2003, p. C3.
[30] *Ibid.*

According to the SARS Expert Committee Report released on October 2, there was no individual "culpable of negligence, lack of diligence or maladministration in the handling of the SARS epidemic". However, it was noted that Hong Kong hospitals had inadequate surge capacity, i.e., limited ability to handle a sudden influx of patients. It was recommended that there be more investment in isolation rooms, and infectious disease units attached to various acute care wards. Plans needed to be put in place which indicated how, in the event of a similar incident, resources would be shared with no one part of the health system becoming overwhelmed.

A "better partnership" was recommended between the public and private health sectors to cope with future public health emergencies. It was apparent that despite the critical nature of the crisis, the public Hospital Authority (HA), for financial reasons, was reluctant to transfer patients to the private hospitals; that private practitioners were not given accurate information from the HA, and had difficulty securing supplies of protection equipment because it was competing for them with the HA.

Like their counterparts everywhere in the world, Hong Kong's medical professionals were frustrated by their lack of knowledge. Weeks went by when there was great uncertainty over how the virus was being transmitted. However, Hong Kong's health workers distinguished themselves by remaining on duty. By contrast, many doctors and nurses in Taipei quit or did not come to work, saying they did not want to expose themselves to the disease.

The government of Hong Kong was also relatively transparent. Much to its credit, it did not try to cover up the outbreak as did the mainland government. As Christine Loh, founder of the Hong Kong public interest group Civic Exchange noted: "Once the Hong Kong government knew it had a problem, it opened up. In China, the instinct was to close down."[31] She and Hong Kong General Chamber of Commerce Eden Woon emphasized that the crisis showed Hong Kong's strengths. Although the Hong Kong government was initially slow to respond to SARS, once mobilized, together with the media, in sharp contrast with

[31] Mark Clifford. "Hong Kong's moment of truth", *Business Week Online*, 26 Jun 2003 (13 Sept 2003).

the response of China's Communist Party rulers in Beijing, it tried to solve the problem openly and with a strong sense of civic responsibility.[32]

Indeed, Hong Kong society in general, though already disappointed with the government's performance before the outbreak, and again disheartened by the delayed response to this new challenge, collaborated closely and efficiently with the government throughout the episode. Besides instituting strong legal and educational systems, the British had fostered innumerable religious and civic organizations which served to act as bridges between individuals, businesses and the government. It had always been generally recognized that the government could not always meet every need in society, and that people needed to form their own small groups to provide immediate, compassionate assistance. Related to this, under the British, Hong Kong always enjoyed a relatively free press.

In urban and rural communities around the world, the formation of civil society organizations (CSOs) — community-based organizations, non-governmental organizations (NGOs), indigenous peoples organizations, labor unions, faith-based groups, professional associations, universities, and foundations — is increasingly regarded as an effective way to reduce human suffering of any kind. They typically foster public-private cooperation, contribute local knowledge and innovative ideas, provide technical expertise, and leverage social capital. In so doing, they contribute to governments' transparency and accountability, and policy and program formulation. They provide a counterweight to state power and provide a venue for the powerless to assert their rights.

Pivotal in reducing the impact of the SARS crisis were the activities and events of over 1,000 Hong Kong CSOs. For example, "Operation UNITE" was established on March 25. By May, some 5,000 volunteers had enlisted and were divided into three teams: educational, support, and caring.[33] The Department of Health assisted the members of the educational team distribute 370,000 leaflets relating to SARS prevention at railway stations, ports and residential areas. Other members of this team set up information booths in public housing areas and handed out SARS

[32] *Ibid*.

[33] "Hong Kong volunteers help fight SARS", 14 May 2003 on World Volunteer Web at http://www.worldvolunteerweb.org, Oct 2003.

prevention kits to elderly people. Others assisted the Home Affairs Department in informing residents of 18 districts on how to avoid SARS.

The support team raised funds and worked with the Red Cross in assembling SARS prevention kits. Volunteers from the Federation of Medical Societies of Hong Kong and the Hong Kong College of Nursing conducted free seminars for the campaign.

Other volunteers systematically telephoned the homes of the elderly and poor and provided information on ways to avoid SARS. This campaign also encouraged NGOs and the general public to contact infected people and offer support. Other volunteers cleaned the homes of elderly people.

Amongst many other examples of organizations immediately offering their services during the crisis were several groups which raised funds. The "Hong Kong is Our Home" Group united more than 600 different community organizations and raised HK$5 million (US$643,848) specifically to express gratitude to the frontline medical and healthcare workers. In only one day, the "Business Community Relief Fund for Victims of SARS", established by the industrial and commercial sectors, raised HK$17 million (US$2.19 million) for SARS victims.

The "'We Care' Education Fund", established by four senior female government officers raised HK$76 million (US$9.79 million), and the "Project Blossom" and "1:99 Charity Concert" together raised another HK$18 million (US$2.32 million), all to be devoted to educational assistance for children who had lost their parents to SARS.

According to a survey conducted by the New Territories Association of Societies in Hong Kong in which 829 people were randomly contacted by phone, 63% of Hong Kong people were willing to provide help to their neighbors if the latter needed to be quarantined, and 65% said Hong Kong's various walks of life had demonstrated their potential unity.[34]

Conclusion

In order to manage future SARS-type crises, governments around the world, including Hong Kong's, have recognized the fact that relevant gov-

[34] "Hong Kong people show unity after SARS outbreak: Survey", *People's Daily Online*, 14 May 2003.

ernment departments must have the structures in place to issue warnings as well as timely, accurate, and reliable detailed information to the public on short notice, and mobilize financial and social resources quickly.

Though the public was once again dissatisfied with the government's behavior, and rejected the final report of the experts commissioned to review the handling of the outbreak, it recognized that Hong Kong's healthcare system stood up comparatively well.[35] All in all, it managed better than Taiwan's and Canada's.

However, the response of Hong Kong's CSOs and the public was crucial. Though greatly disillusioned with the government long before SARS struck, many existing non-governmental organizations, which had successfully bridged individuals, businesses and the government for decades, played a key role in halting the spread of the disease and reducing fear, confusion and near hysteria at every level of society. Moreover, new volunteer organizations sprang into existence to deal specifically with controlling the disease.

On one hand, the SARS crisis accentuated the problems of the government. It highlighted some difficulties in the Territory's political leadership, as well as shortfalls in the adaptability of the bureaucracy, and overall transparency and accountability of the system. On the other, it brought people together in civil society. It fostered a sense of solidarity and forced them, more than ever, to learn how to co-operate, possibly creating new political structures for moving forward out of the increasingly bitter political malaise that the Territory had been in since 1997.

It is impossible to know whether or not the number of people infected by SARS in Hong Kong would have been less had there been a more democratic form of government. Some poor judgement calls, resulting mainly from a lack of knowledge about the disease, would likely have occurred regardless of the type of government system. However, perhaps it can be said that the performance of Hong Kong's civil society outshone that of the government, providing further proof that executive-led, top-down planning is not necessary, and may indeed be detrimental to Hong Kong's best interests.

[35] "Hong Kong SARS whitewash", *Asian Wall Street Journal*, 7 Oct 1993.

Index

60 SARS patients and seven had already died in a military hospital. The Chinese media did not dare publish Dr. Jiang's letter. It was the *Time* magazine which finally released the true information as told by Dr. Jiang on April 8, 2003.[21] While SARS patients in No. 301 military hospital were not under the Ministry of Health's purview due to the bifurcation of military-civilian authority, "the PLA's poor record in revealing information to civilian authorities in the early days of the SARS outbreak can be attributed to the sense of autonomy and secrecy that has long characterized the military in China".[22]

Originally, SARS was regarded as a local medical issue in February and March 2003. When it became a regional epidemic, it was deemed as a political issue in April 2003. On April 7 Premier Wen Jiabao visited China's Center for Disease Control and talked about the PLA's failure to report on the SARS outbreak.[23] A special Politburo meeting was held on April 17. On April 20, the Politburo Standing Committee warned against the covering up of SARS cases and demanded the accurate, timely, and honest reporting of the SARS situation. Minister of Health Zhang Wenkang and Beijing Mayor Meng Xuenong were sacked on April 20. A National Task Force headed by Wu Yi was established. On July 24, 2003, the World Health Organization (WHO) lifted a travel advisory it had issued against Beijing.

It should be stressed that the change in Chinese government's attitude was largely due to international pressure and globalization of the disease. Wu Guoguang, a professor at the Chinese University of Hong Kong, commented: "In the past, lies did harm only to the Chinese. Those who were killed as a result of lies did not know what actually happened. At present, a single lie told by China will throw the whole world into panic, as if the world is faced with a formidable enemy."[24] The SARS disease has spread to at least 28 countries including Australia, Brazil, Canada, South Africa, Spain, and the United States. The number of probable cases reached 8098 worldwide by July 31, 2003 (see Table 2). As Zhang Erping

[21] Susan Jakes. "Beijing's SARS attack: Doctor and party member insist there are many more cases than officials will admit", *Time*, 8 Apr 2003.

[22] Joseph Fewsmith. "China and the politics of SARS", p. 253.

[23] *Ibid.*, p. 250.

[24] Wu Guoguang. "How to test the truth of speeches", *Hsin Pao*, Hong Kong, 29 Apr 2003.

Table 2. Summary of Probable SARS Cases with Onset of Illness from November 1, 2002 to July 31, 2003 (Revised September 26, 2003)

	Cumulative number of cases									
Areas	F	M	Total of cases	Median age (range)	Number of deaths	Case fatality ratio (%)	Number of imported case (%)	Number of HCW affected (%)	Date onset first probable case	Date onset last probable case
Canada	151	100	251	49(1–45)	43	17	5 (2)	109(43)	23-Feb-03	12-Jun-03
China (PRC)	2674	2607	5327	Pending	349	7	Not applicable	1002(19)	16-Nov-02	3-Jun-03
China, Hong Kong	977	778	1755	40(1–100)	299	17	Not applicable	386(22)	15-Feb-03	31-May-03
China, Macao	0	1	1	28	0	0	1(100)	0(0)	5-May-03	5-May-03
China, Taiwan	218	128	346	42(0–93)	37	11	21(6)	68(20)	25-Feb-03	15-Jun-03
Singapore	161	77	238	35(1–90)	33	14	8(3)	97(41)	25-Feb-03	5-May-03
Vietnam	39	24	63	43(20–76)	5	5	1(2)	36(57)	23-Feb-03	14-Apr-03

Source: http://www.who.int/csr/sars/country/table2003_09_23/en/, accessed on 18 Feb 2004.